Ciba Foundation
Study Group No. 31

NUTRITION AND INFECTION

Ciba Foundation
Study Group
No. 31

Nutrition
and Infection

In honour of   Professor R. Nicolaysen

Edited by   G. E. W. Wolstenholme
and
Maeve O'Connor

With 20 Illustrations

1967

J. & A. CHURCHILL LTD.
104 GLOUCESTER PLACE
LONDON, W.I

Standard Book Number
7000 1344 X

Printed in Great Britain

23.1.68

The Ciba Foundation

 The Ciba Foundation was opened in 1949 to promote international co-operation in medical and chemical research among scientists from all parts of the world. Its house at 41 Portland Place, London, has become a meeting place well known to workers in many fields of science. Every year the Foundation organizes from six to ten three-day symposia and three or four one-day study groups, all of which are published in book form. Many other informal meetings also take place in the house, organized either by the Foundation or by other scientific groups needing a place to meet. In addition, bedrooms are available for visiting scientists, whether or not they are attending a meeting in the building.

The Ciba Foundation owes its existence to the generosity of CIBA Ltd, Basle, who, realizing the disruption of scientific communication caused by the war and by problems of distance, decided to set up a philanthropic institution whose aim would be to overcome such barriers. London was chosen as its site for reasons dictated by the special advantages of English charitable trust law, as well as those of language and geography.

The Foundation's many activities are controlled by a small group of distinguished trustees. Within the general framework of biological science, interpreted in its broadest sense, these activities are well summed up by the Ciba Foundation's motto, *Consocient Gentes*—let the nations come together.

Contents

Membership
Study Group on Nutrition and Infection held
8th June, 1967

W. R. Aykroyd	. .	Queen Anne House, Church Lane, Charlbury, Oxfordshire
W. T. C. Berry	. .	Ministry of Health, London
J. F. Brock.	. .	Department of Medicine, Wernher and Beit Medical Laboratories, University of Cape Town
N. T. A. Byam	. .	Trinidad Nutritional Centre, Trinidad
M. A. Crawford	. .	Nuffield Institute of Comparative Medicine, Zoological Society of London
Wenche B. Eide	.	Institute of Nutrition Research, University of Oslo
J. S. Garrow*	. .	MRC Tropical Metabolism Research Unit, St. Mary's Hospital, London
B. E. Gustafsson	.	Department of Germfree Research, Karolinska Institutet, Stockholm
+P. György	. .	Department of Public Health, Phila- delphia General Hospital, Philadelphia
R. G. Hendrickse	.	Department of Paediatrics, University of Ibadan
D. B. Jelliffe	. .	Caribbean Food and Nutrition Institute, University of the West Indies, Jamaica
E. F. Patricia Jelliffe.		Caribbean Food and Nutrition Institute, University of the West Indies, Jamaica
H. A. M. Khan	. .	School of Paediatrics, Jinnah Post- graduate Medical Centre, Karachi
E. Kodicek	. .	Dunn Nutritional Laboratory, Uni- versity of Cambridge and MRC, Cambridge
B. G. Maegraith	.	Department of Tropical Medicine, Liverpool School of Tropical Medicine
L. J. Mata	. .	Institute of Nutrition of Central America and Panama, Guatemala

* Present adress: Department of Obstetrics and Gynaecology,
Royal Free Hospital, Liverpool Road, London
+Unable to attend.

D. C. Morley	.	.	Institute of Child Health, University of London
R. Nicolaysen	.	.	Institute for Nutrition Research, University of Oslo
J. I. Pedersen	.	.	Institute for Nutrition Research, University of Oslo
H. M. Sinclair	.	.	Magdalen College, Oxford
B. Vahlquist	.	.	Department of Paediatrics, University Hospital, Uppsala
W. Wittman .	.	.	National Nutrition Research Institute of the CSIR, Pretoria
Sir Norman Wright		.	British Association for the Advancement of Science, London

CHAIRMAN'S INTRODUCTION

PROFESSOR J. F. BROCK

I am very happy to be chairman of this study group on Nutrition and Infection, firstly because it is organized by the Ciba Foundation, whose standing in the field of advancement and critical assessment of biomedical research is so high, and secondly because it is held in honour of one whose work has for many years commanded my respect.

Ragnar Nicolaysen's work first came to my attention when I was receiving my own introduction to medical research in the field of parathyroid glands and bone diseases at the London Hospital. In 1932 he published three papers (Nicolaysen, R. [1932]. *Biochem. Z.*, **248**, 275-277; **248**, 278-279; Jervell, O., and Nicolaysen, R. [1932]. *Biochem. Z.*, **250**, 308-311), all of which were concerned with calcium and he has confirmed to me that these were his first scientific papers.

His continuing interest in the physiology of calcium metabolism is evident in his review under this heading in 1953 (Nicolaysen, R., Eeg-Larsen, N., and Malm, O. J. [1953]. *Physiol. Rev.*, **33**, 424-444). Special aspects of this general interest are evident in his review (with N. Eeg-Larsen) of the biochemistry and physiology of Vitamin D in volume 11 (1953, pp. 29-60) of *Vitamins and Hormones*, and communications to the first *Ciba Foundation Colloquium on Ageing* (1955. *General Aspects*) and the *Ciba Foundation Symposium on Bone Structure and Metabolism* (1956). These four reviews epitomize an interest in calcium which evolved from his initial studies in 1932 and are the fruit of a quarter of a century of scientific study, experiment and reflection.

1

As his scientific life has matured Professor Nicolaysen has been drawn, both by inner conviction and by the pressure of national responsibility, into concern for the application of advances in the science of nutrition and metabolism to human welfare. As one who has gone through a somewhat similar evolution I can understand both the conflict of interest which plagues and the inward satisfactions which relieve the process.

For the last decade or more the focus of his nutritional interest has moved steadily into the field of what he calls nutrition in a welfare state, or the effects on health of dietary self-selection in a privileged community. He has concerned himself with advancing knowledge of over-nutrition in general and in particular of the relationships between quantity and quality of dietary fats and the evolution of atherosclerosis and its complications.

His growing reputation as an adviser in public health nutrition and in the development of research policy in his university and in national institutions and councils has brought a sense of responsibility for the difficult decisions which have to be made in the face of public excitement about half-baked theories on diet and health. This in turn has led to his great interest in the foundation of an institute for the graduate training of nutrition workers which he hopes will serve the Scandinavian countries and which has become the focus of his thought and work.

Ragnar Nicolaysen's gifts and his contributions to science have been recognized in his election to numerous offices in the councils and academies of his country. Norway and Oslo can be proud of a Norwegian who through a lifetime·of hard work has brought lustre to his nation.

INTRODUCTION OF SPECIFIC MICRO-ORGANISMS INTO GERM-FREE ANIMALS

BENGT E. GUSTAFSSON

Department of Germfree Research, Karolinska Institutet, Stockholm

The absence of the normal indigenous microbial flora is followed by specific anatomical and physiological alterations or symptoms in germ-free animals, in comparison with conventional animals reared on the same diet (for surveys see Mickelsen, 1962; Luckey, 1963). More than 20 such symptoms have so far been described, including an enlarged caecum and reduced lymphoid tissue with a low γ-globulin content in the serum. The faeces of germ-free animals contains unchanged bile acids and cholesterol but no coprostanol, bilirubin but no urobilin, and also active digestive enzymes, like trypsin, which are lacking in the conventional animals. Germ-free animals can also develop deficiencies of vitamins, which are normally produced by intestinal micro-organisms.

All these symptoms are compensated by the introduction of so-called normal intestinal flora from conventional animals. The question may arise of whether specific micro-organisms are necessary or whether this compensation of the germ-free symptoms is mediated by the presence of a great number of strains which can substitute for each other. In the former case the situation in mammals, including man, would be similar to the endosymbiosis between micro-organisms and host organisms which is so common in insects, where the presence of highly specified micro-organisms is necessary for the normal life of the host. The endosymbionts in insects usually produce vitamins or are effective in the digestion, for example of cellulose, as is

3

the case in termites. The interaction with certain highly
specialized micro-organisms in the rumen of ruminants
which occurs in the digestion of cellulose might also be
labelled endosymbiosis.

CONTAMINATION WITH FULL FLORA

As germ-free animals have an underdeveloped lymphatic
system and low γ-globulin and properdin levels in their
sera, the transformation from the germ-free to the
conventional state might be expected to be somewhat
difficult. When germ-free rats are transferred from the

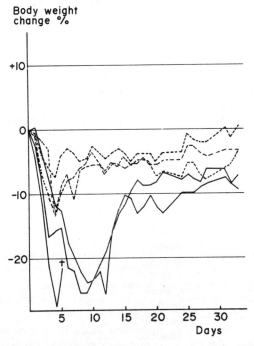

Fig. 1. Weight changes of germ-free rats transferred to the animal
room, infected at random (—) or given an enema of caecum contents
from conventional animals (- - -).

germ-free isolator to separate cages in the animal room so that they are open to infection from any micro-organisms that are present, they usually show severe diarrhoea and a sharp drop in weight lasting several weeks. Occasionally these animals die (Fig. 1). When their germ-free litter-mates are similarly kept in separate cages in the animal room but given an enema with a suspension of caecum contents from conventional rats, there is no diarrhoea, only a slight drop in weight, and no deaths. As would be expected, mice are more susceptible than rats (Table I), but a greater number of them die when they are infected at random. Feeding caecum contents of conventional animals

Table I

CONTAMINATION OF GERM-FREE MICE WITH CAECUM
CONTENTS OF CONVENTIONAL ANIMALS

Housing during contamination	Mode of contamination	Number of animals		
		Total	With diarrhoea	Dead
Animal room, separate cages	In feed	40	9	5
	Accidental	36	20	14
GF isolator, separate cages	In feed	34	0	0
	Accidental	33	19	4

to germ-free mice kept in the isolator has a protective effect, whereas litter-mates in separate cages in the same isolator, which pick up contaminants from the caecal contents only from the air or through contact with the gloves of the operator, show diarrhoea, and deaths occur.

The diarrhoea and deaths among these random-infected animals during "conventionalization" must be caused by micro-organisms, the exact nature of which is still being investigated. Up to now it has not been possible to connect any specific type of micro-organism with the transmission syndrome. It is, however, interesting to note

that when *Clostridium difficile* is introduced into mice and
rats a similar condition may appear. Skelly, Trexler and
Tanami (1962) isolated from conventional mice a bacterium
which reduced the enlarged caeca, and they classified the
organism as a strain of *Clostridium difficile*. When an
American Type Culture Collection strain of this organism
was fed in our laboratory to germ-free mice, only seven out
of 78 animals exposed survived. On the other hand, when
germ-free animals that had been infected with caecum
contents 14 days previously received *Clostridium difficile*,
no diarrhoea or deaths occurred (Table II).

Table II

INTRODUCTION OF *CLOSTRIDIUM DIFFICILE* INTO GERM-FREE MICE

	Number of Animals		
Nature of contaminant	Total	*With diarrhoea*	*Dead*
Original strain	78	78	71
Caecum contents from conventional mice + original strain after 14 days	28	0	0

THE ACTION OF SPECIFIC MICRO-ORGANISMS IN VITAMIN K-DEFICIENT ANIMALS

Growth and reproduction is normal in animals on a
semi-synthetic diet containing all the known vitamins,
including vitamin K. Our germ-free strain of rats was
created by Caesarean section in 1956 and has now reached
the 25th inbred generation on the same semi-synthetic diet
(Table III) (Gustafsson, 1959a). When the casein and wheat
starch is extracted with light petroleum and vitamin K is
omitted from this diet, however, all the germ-free animals

die within a few weeks with extensive haemorrhages and a
very low prothrombin content in the blood (Gustafsson,
1959b; Gustafsson et al., 1952). When such animals, highly
deficient in vitamin K and with prothrombin levels below
10 per cent, were removed from the germ-free isolators to a
cage which was heavily smeared with faeces from normal
animals, the deficient animals recovered within 24 hours,
whereas an animal put into a sterilized glass jar in an
ordinary laboratory room did not show any real recovery
within 48 hours (Fig. 2). By infecting a series of

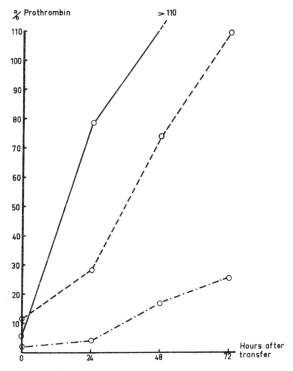

Fig. 2. Prothrombin values in germ-free rats with vitamin K
deficiency transferred to a heavily infected ordinary cage (o—o):
to a moderately infected metabolism cage (o----o); and isolated
in glass jars in the laboratory (o-·-·o). (From Gustafsson, 1959b).

Table III

COMPOSITION OF DIET D7

Casein	22%
Wheat starch	63%
Arachis oil	10%
Salt mixture HMW*	4%
Vitamin mixtures	1%
Vitamins added per 100 g. diet:	
Vitamin A	2100 i.u.
Vitamin D	450 i.u.
Vitamin E	50 mg.
Vitamin K	1 mg.
Thiamine	5 mg.
Riboflavin	2 mg.
Pyridoxine	2 mg.
Calcium pantothenate	10 mg.
Nicotinamide	20 mg.
Choline	200 mg.
Inositol	100 mg.
p-Aminobenzoic acid	30 mg.
Biotin	0·1 mg.
Folic acid	2 mg.
Vitamin B_{12}	0·002 mg.
Ascorbic acid	100 mg.

* Hubbell, Mendel and Wakeman (1937).

germ-free rats which were housed separately in isolators, we were able to demonstrate that the vitamin K deficiency could be alleviated by the introduction of certain bacteria (Table IV), one of which was highly active, belonging to genera found in the intestinal tract or in the mouth of conventional rats.

UROBILIN FORMATION IN MONOCONTAMINATED AND DI-CONTAMINATED RATS

No urobilinogens are present in the faeces or urine of germ-free rats (Gustafsson and Lanke, 1960). After contamination of the germ-free rats with faeces from conventional animals, the production of urobilins was already, on the third day after contamination, of about the

same magnitude as in conventional rats. From the
intestinal contents of one of the ex-germ-free rats a
clostridium-like organism (G 62) was isolated. After this
bacterium had been established in germ-free rats, the tests
for urobilins in faeces became positive on the second or third
day. The quantity of urobilins produced in 24 hours was,
however, low in comparison with that in the conventional
rats.

Table IV

EFFECT OF MONOCONTAMINATIONS IN SINGLE VITAMIN K-DEFICIENT GERM-FREE RATS

(from Gustafsson *et al.*, 1962)

Type of micro-organism*	Source	Prothrombin activity values after 48 hours †
		%
Sarcina	Rat oral and enteric strain	100
Escherichia coli	Rat enteric strain	100
Lactobacillus acidophilus	Rat oral strain	< 10
Diphtheroid	Rat oral strain	< 10
Sporeformer	Rat enteric strain	< 10
Bacteroides I	Rat enteric strain	< 10
Bacteroides II	Rat enteric strain	< 10
None	—	< 10

*Each animal received the equivalent of 0·1 ml. of a 24-hour
broth culture which was washed and resuspended in saline.
†Initial prothrombin activity < 10%.

When germ-free animals were again infected with the same
strain of *Clostridium* (G 62) and with a strain of *E. coli*
(G 14), the animals produced more urobilins than the rats
infected with *Clostridium* (G 62) only (Table V). But on the
15th to 18th day after infection the urobilin content in the
faeces was still only about a third of that in conventional
rats.

Several known strains of bacteria were also tested and
proved to have no effect on urobilin formation. The bacteria

tested were: *Clostridium welchii* type A, alone or in
combination with strains of *E. coli* of human origin, *E. coli*
alone, *Enterococcus* alone or in combination with *E. coli* of
rat origin (G 14), *Clostridium sporogenes* alone,
Lactobacillus acidophilus alone, *Proteus vulgaris* alone,
and strains of *B. subtilis*, *Sarcina* and *Mucor*.

Table V

UROBILINS IN FAECES FROM EX-GERM-FREE RATS CONTAMINATED
WITH *CLOSTRIDIUM* (G 62) OR WITH *CLOSTRIDIUM* (G 62)
+ *E. COLI* (G 14)

(from Gustafsson and Lanke, 1960)

(Urobilins calculated as micromoles of stercobilinogen per kilogram
body weight per 24 hours)

Animal No.	Contaminated with	Days after contamination 112—115					
5	*Clostridium* (G 62)	0·12	0·11	0·11	0·34		
6	*Clostridium* (G 62)	0·17	0·08	0·11	0·32		
7	*Clostridium* (G 62)	0·27	0·15	0·34	0·25	0·72	0·25
8	*Clostridium* (G 62) + *E. coli* (G 14)	0·52	0·86	0·77	1·34		
9	*Clostridium* (G 62) + *E. coli* (G 14)	0·30	0·37	0·91	0·89		
10	*Clostridium* (G 62) + *E. coli* (G 14)	0·82	0·79	0·99	0·94		

ESTABLISHMENT OF DECONJUGATING AND
7α-DEHYDROXYLATING MICRO-ORGANISMS IN GERM-FREE
RATS

Deconjugation of the primary bile acids and the formation
of lithocholic acid are the main features of the metabolism
of bile acids in conventional rats. These reactions are
absent in the germ-free rat, where the primary conjugated
bile acids are secreted in the faeces. Several strains of
intestinal bacteria are able to deconjugate, but so far only
one group of organisms isolated from rat and human faeces

is capable of 7α-dehydroxylating the bile acids (Gustafsson, Midtvedt and Norman, 1966). These organisms have been identified by Midtvedt (1967) as anaerobic members of the tribe *Lactobacillus*. One of these organisms, labelled strain II, was further studied in monocontamination experiments. Although this organism was isolated from conventional rats, it proved rather difficult to establish as

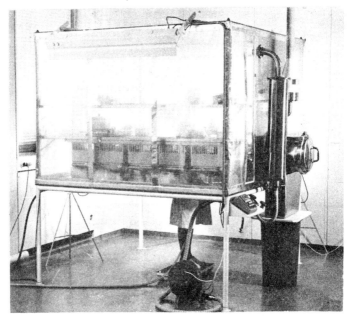

Fig. 3a. A jacket isolator used in contamination studies.

a monocontaminant in germ-free animals. It was easily established, however, with both deconjugating and non-conjugating bacteria in large numbers, i.e. 10^9-10^{10}/g. faeces (Gustafsson, Midtvedt and Norman, 1967). But when radioactively labelled cholic acid was administered much less of it transformed to its various metabolites than was found in conventional rats on the same diet (Gustafsson and Norman, 1962).

The difficulty of getting strain II established is also demonstrated by the following experiment (Gustafsson, Midtvedt and Norman, 1967). One rat (no. 6 in Fig. 3*b*), harbouring strain II, was brought into a large (6×6 feet) jacket isolator on the same side as three other rats, two of which (nos. 11 and 13) were contaminated with faeces from

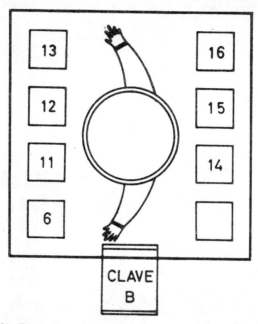

Fig. 3b. Plan of isolator with metabolism cages. Numbers refer to animals in Fig. 4. (From Gustafsson, Midtvedt and Norman, 1967.)

rat no. 6. Strain II became established in both these and no. 12 (Fig. 4). On the other hand, two animals (nos. 14 and 16) infected with a broth culture of strain II, and the control animal on the same side, remained germ-free for five months, although these animals had to be handled by the same attendant as those in which strain II was established with the faecal culture.

Close physical contact between two animals seems to be necessary, as well as factors hitherto not very well known, for the establishment and normal action in the animals of these physiologically important micro-organisms.

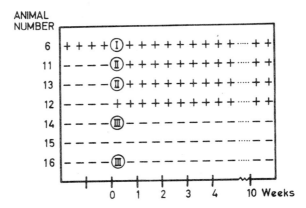

Fig. 4. Contamination of germ-free rats in an isolator with strain II. Animals nos. 11, 13, 14 and 16 were voluntarily contaminated with

   I = Strain II in a previous experiment;
   II = Faeces from rat no. 6;
   III = A 7-day-old culture of strain II in Todd Hewitt (Oxoid) broth.

Subcultures of faeces were made twice a week. −: no growth, +: growth of Strain II. (From Gustafsson, Midtvedt and Norman, 1967.)

SUMMARY

With the exception of the demonstrated effect of vitamin-producing bacteria, very few, if any, germ-free characteristics have been fully compensated by the introduction into germ-free animals of specific micro-organisms. Strain II, for example, fully 7α-dehydroxylates bile acids *in vitro*, but less than 10 per cent is 7α-dehydroxylated *in vivo*. Despite much work by ourselves

and others, nobody has been able permanently to reduce the
enlarged caecum with single strains of micro-organisms.
The outcome of the work on the urobilinogen-forming and
bile-acid-metabolizing bacteria seems to warrant the
conclusion that association with a second or third micro-
organism is necessary for the full effect of the pertinent
organism.

The final goal of these studies on the establishment in
germ-free animals of physiologically important micro-organisms is to determine the members of what could be termed
the minimal essential indigenous flora. The work so far
shows that we are dealing with rather fastidious unclassified micro-organisms which are not easily handled either
in the laboratory or in animal experiments.

Interactions between these bacteria and the host, and
among the bacteria themselves, cannot, however, be
excluded when the nutrition and infection of higher animals
and man is considered.

REFERENCES

Gustafsson, B. E. (1959a). *Ann. N.Y. Acad. Sci.*, **78**, 17-28.
Gustafsson, B. E. (1959b). *Ann. N.Y. Acad. Sci.*, **78**, 166-173.
Gustafsson, B. E., Daft, F. S., McDaniel, E. G., Smith, J. C.,
and Fitzgerald, R. J. (1962). *J. Nutr.*, **78**, 461-468.
Gustafsson, B. E., and Lanke, L. Swenander (1960). *J. exp. Med.*,
112, 975-981.
Gustafsson, B. E., Midtvedt, T., and Norman, A. (1966). *J. exp.
Med.*, **123**, 413-432.
Gustafsson, B. E., Midtvedt, T., and Norman, A. (1967). *Acta
path. microbiol. scand.*, in press.
Gustafsson, B. E., and Norman, A. (1962). *Proc. Soc. exp. Biol.
Med.*, **110**, 387-389.
Hubbell, R. B., Mendel, L. B., and Wakeman, A. J. (1937).
J. Nutr., **14**, 273-285.
Luckey, T. D. (1963). *Germfree Life and Gnotobiology*. New York
and London: Academic Press.
Midtvedt, T. (1967). *Acta path. microbiol. scand.*, in press.
Mickelsen, O. (1962). *A. Rev. Biochem.*, **31**, 515-548.
Skelly, B. J., Trexler, P. C., and Tanami, J. (1962). *Proc. Soc.
Exp. Biol. Med.*, **110**, 455-458.

DISCUSSION

Maegraith: Can you tell us something about the absorption of foodstuffs in the small intestine in these germ-free animals, Professor Gustafsson? Disturbance of the bacterial content of the small intestine may be connected with the malabsorption which occurs in sprue, for example. This may also involve the independent anaerobes: have you seen any such organisms?

Gustafsson: There is some evidence that the absence of the flora influences the absorption rate of amino acids and minerals. As to the numbers and types of organisms present in the intestines, one must remember that more than 50 per cent of the microbial strains inhabiting the gut are very little known and are unclassified.

Jelliffe: Your paper has immense relevance for those of us who work in tropical countries, Professor Gustafsson. Although our environments are far from germ-free, I would like to suggest that both travellers' diarrhoea and that major scourge associated with malnutrition—weanling diarrhoea—are both very possibly due, in part, to what one might call "germ-change", which is surely part of your thesis.

Mata: The contamination of the human newborn, which is virtually a germ-free animal at the moment of birth, is now of interest to INCAP workers. From our studies of village children, we know that the flora of one child may be different from that of another child of the same age living in the same house. If both children are exposed to the same bacterium, only one of them may get infected with it. This phenomenon of bacterial interference, which has been called infection-immunity (Dubos, R. [1963]. *Am. J. Dis. Child.*, **105**, 643), has been demonstrated for the microbiota of the skin and other sites of the body (Hurst, V. [1965]. In *Skin Bacteria and Their Role in Infection*, pp. 127-141, ed. Maibach, H. I., and Hildick-Smith, G. New York: McGraw-Hill; Shinefield, H. R., Ribble, J. C., Boris, M., and Eichenwald, H. F. [1963]. *Am. J. Dis. Child.*, **105**, 646). Recently, some workers have reported on the feasibility of establishing one type of *E. coli* in the intestine at birth (Lodinova, R., Jouja, V., and Lanc, A. [1967]. *J. Bact.*, **93**, 797). Undoubtedly, this method of putting germs back into germ-free animals has great relevance for the human host, but we must find out first how the human intestinal tract is colonized, because we know nothing about this basic phenomenon.

Crawford: The other side of the germ-free problem is germ excess. In East Africa people living on a staple diet of plantains or sweet potatoes, which are low in tryptophan, excrete large quantities of bacterial degradation products of tryptophan, which is quite surprising. One possible explanation is that such diets lead to increased small gut motility which passes the tryptophan down to the bacteria, so that an excessive and prolonged excretion occurs of both indican. a normal bacterial metabolite of tryptophan, and an unusual bacterial metabolite of tryptophan, namely indolyl acrylic acid and its glycine conjugate (Banwell, J., and Crawford, M. A. [1963]. *Biochem. J.*, 89, 69-70; Crawford, M. A. [1964]. *E. Afr. med. J.*, 41, 228-238). These bacterial products are associated with diet, being present in the urine of plantain/sweet potato eaters but not in those existing on maize or milk diets. Neomycin can be used to suppress the bacterial responses to a tryptophan load.

The question that arises is whether excessive bacterial degradation in these plantain/sweet potato eaters means that these people are losing significant quantities of essential amino acids in this way.

Professor Gustafsson noticed that trypsin was present in the faeces of the germ-free animals. Is it present because the bacteria under normal circumstances stop digestion by inactivating the enzymes, or are the bacteria themselves contributing to the nitrogen balance in the host? We know from comparative studies that in the ruminant, the bacteria synthesize amino acids from dietary nitrogen. In the pseudo-ruminant the story is halfway between exogenous protein and endogenous synthesis by the flora. In man we apparently know absolutely nothing about what happens, although we are beginning to learn something from these germ-free studies.

Kodicek: If there is a reduction of the tryptophan intake by bacterial degradation, do people on a plantain or sweet potato diet show signs of nicotinic acid deficiency? One would expect that tryptophan is the main source of nicotinic acid in these diets.

Crawford: As far as I know, no gross signs of nicotinic acid deficiency appear. An almost identical but more severe urinary pattern is seen in Hartnup disease in response to a tryptophan load. However, we know this is due neither to increased bacteria nor increased motility but to a failure in the enzyme transport system of the small gut; a photosensitive pellagra is characteristic.

Gustafsson: Our theory at present is that digestive enzymes in the normal intestine are inactivated by bacteria, as we have demonstrated for trypsin.

The question of protein synthesis by the bacteria in the gut is very complicated. If germ-free and conventional animals are put on a protein-limited diet, such as a 6-8 per cent casein diet, the germ-free animals continue to grow when the others have stopped.

The implication is of course that the normal flora uses part of the protein intake. Recently, however, this situation has become more complicated by the finding that some of the bacteria in the gut are digested while some are not (data not yet published). So in the conventional animal it is also a question of what kind of flora they have: if they have the type of flora which is digested, the loss of nitrogen due to the presence of the flora is less than if they have the type of flora which is not digested.

PLACENTAL MALARIA AND FOETAL GROWTH FAILURE

E. F. Patricia Jelliffe

Department of Paediatrics, Makerere Medical School, Kampala, Uganda*

The possible ill effects of placental malaria on neonatal development were first noted by Clarke in 1915, working in Panama. Since then 15 or more studies have been carried out, the main emphasis being directed towards the malarial picture in indigenous African women. In different areas of Nigeria, Bruce-Chwatt (1952), Archibald (1956, 1958), Cannon (1958), and Spitz (1959) found that mothers with infected placentae gave birth in all instances to smaller infants, the difference in mean birth weight varying from 89 g. to as much as 312 g. In East Africa, McLaren and Ward (1962) stressed in their study the importance of considering the birth rank and sex of the neonates.

Despite their importance and relevance to the continuous problem of infant wastage in developing countries, the impact of these studies on practising obstetricians and paediatricians appears to have been slight, and this cause of low birth weight is rarely mentioned in paediatric textbooks. This apparent indifference in countries in which malaria exists endemically could be attributed to a lack of awareness of this problem on the part of the medical staff, an overwhelming burden of routine work, insufficient channels for dissemination of knowledge between adjoining African territories, lack of laboratory and research personnel, and general paucity of governmental finances to alleviate this unnecessary cause of low birth weight.

*Present address: Caribbean Food and Nutrition Institute, University of the West Indies, Jamaica.

The task of collecting placentae, and ascertaining that the rightful owner and corresponding baby are found, can be tedious, difficult and time-consuming in a large understaffed maternity centre, but it is the essential focal point of these studies, as a negative maternal peripheral blood does not exclude placental malaria.

METHOD OF STUDY

The present study was undertaken in Kampala, Uganda during two separate periods of six consecutive months, each covering both wet and dry seasons. Five hundred and seventy women, their placentae and singleton live-born neonates were seen.

These women belonged to as homogeneous a group as possible: all were African women of the lower socioeconomic class—wives of small peasant farmers or slum-dwelling labourers. Sixty-four per cent were Baganda; the remainder belonged to other East African tribal groups. Women who believed they might have received anti-malarial drugs during their pregnancy were excluded from the study. An obstetrical history was taken from each woman and checked with the information collected by the medical officer on the case sheet.

In none of these cases could an accurate gestational period be determined.

BLOOD EXAMINATION

All blood samples were collected between one and 22 hours after delivery. Thick blood films were taken from the peripheral blood of the neonate, cord and mother, and two films were made from the placenta.

ANTHROPOMETRY

All measures were taken on the day of delivery (between one and 22 hours).

(1) *The neonate:*

All infants were weighed by the author on a beam balance scale which was checked daily and at intervals during the day with a series of weights ranging from 4 oz. to 10 lb. (114 g. to 4,450 g.).

If the infants were considered well enough their length was recorded, their head and chest and arm circumferences were taken with a non-stretch tape measure, and the subcutaneous triceps skinfold was recorded with a Harpenden skinfold calliper.

Five hundred and thirty infants were included in this group.

(2) *The mother:*

All mothers were weighed and their height recorded when possible. It was not feasible to disturb women who had undergone surgical intervention, or those with profuse post-partum bleeding or receiving intravenous fluids.

The nutritional status was noted as judged by certain clinical stigmata.

(3) *The placenta:*

All placentae were cleared of clots and carefully examined macroscopically, any abnormalities being noted; 100 placentae were weighed, including membranes and cord.

RESULTS

Of 570 women under consideration, 92 (16·1 per cent) had parasitized placentae and 32 (5·6 per cent) had coincidental infection of the peripheral blood. Only one neonate had a positive blood film (Table I). Infected placentae were observed more frequently (7 per cent) among primiparous women. It was felt that this could be attributed to a lesser degree of immunity to malaria occurring among women of a younger age group.

When the birth weights of the neonates with infected and non-infected placentae were compared, the difference in mean birth weight between the two groups was 263 g. This was statistically highly significant ($P<0.001$) (E. F. P. Jelliffe, 1966) (Table II).

In order to exclude possible genetic differences due to the mixed tribal group, the Baganda and the non-Baganda neonates were considered separately. For both groups a

Table I

INCIDENCE OF MALARIAL INFECTION AMONG 570 AFRICAN WOMEN

Group	Number	+	%.
Mothers	579	32	5.6
Placentae	570	92	16.1
Neonates	569 (1 died 1 hour after birth)	1	0.2

Table II

COMPARATIVE WEIGHTS OF 570 NEONATES IN RELATION TO PLACENTAL MALARIA

Placentae	Number	%.	Mean birth-weight (g.)
Infected	92	16.1	2.805
Non-infected	478	83.9	3.068
Total	570	100.0	3.025
Difference	263 g.	$P = < 0.001$	

lower birth weight was found among the neonates with infected placentae. Among the Baganda babies the mean weight difference was 285 g. and among the non-Baganda 221 g. Both of these results were again statistically highly significant ($P<0.001$).

A higher percentage of neonates with a low birth weight (2,500 g. or below) was also found among the infected

group (19·6 per cent) than among the non-infected group
(10 per cent) (Table III).

Infants born of primiparous mothers are usually lighter in
weight than their subsequent siblings and male infants are

Table III

INCIDENCE OF NEONATES OF LOW BIRTH WEIGHT IN INFECTED
AND NON-INFECTED GROUPS

Neonates of 2,500 g. in weight or less	Infected placentae (92)		Non-infected placentae (478)	
	No.	%	No.	%
Total neonates: 66	18	19·6	48	10·0

Table IV

WEIGHTS OF MALE NEONATES WITH INFECTED AND NON-INFECTED
PLACENTAE BY BIRTH RANK

Birth rank	Infected (g.)	Non-infected (g.)	Difference (g.)
1	2,616 (15)	2,929 (52)	+313
2	2,789 (6)	3,040 (43)	+251
3	2,868 (3)	3,083 (56)	+217
4	2,815 (4)	3,173 (46)	+358
5	3,190 (5)	3,145 (24)	−45*
6	2,849 (8)	3,286 (42)	+437

(−) Indicates number of subjects in group.
(*) In parity 5 the mean birth weight of the non-infected group is
lower than in the infected group.

on the average larger than females. In this study, therefore,
the sex and birth rank of the infants were considered. In
Table IV the male infants are grouped by birth rank, and
except for parity 5 all neonates with infected placentae are

smaller in weight than the non-infected group. Among female neonates (Table V), except for parity 3 the infected group are again smaller in weight than their non-infected counterparts. In the two exceptions noted the increase in mean birth weight among the infected group was small. The

Table V

WEIGHTS OF FEMALE NEONATES WITH INFECTED AND NON-.
INFECTED PLACENTAE BY BIRTH RANK

Birth rank	Infected (g.)	Non-infected (g.)	Difference (g.)
1	2,497 (10)	2,843 (39)	+345
2	2,869 (12)	2,933 (33)	+64
3	3,074 (11)	3,039 (52)	−35*
4	2,790 (8)	3,142 (42)	+352
5	2,978 (3)	3,061 (31)	+83
6	2,721 (7)	3,210 (36)	+489

(−) Denotes the number of subjects in each group.
* In parity 3 the mean birth weight of the non-infected group is lower.

mean birth weight by birth rank showed a constant increase in all ranks from 1 to 4 in both groups, and in both sexes.

The other anthropometric data were as follows:

(a) *Birth length (crown-heel)*

The mean birth length of all infected neonates was reduced (Table VI).

(b) *Head circumference*

Neonates with infected placentae had a smaller head circumference (Table VII).

Table VI

DIFFERENCE IN LENGTH BETWEEN INFECTED AND NON-INFECTED
GROUPS

	Length		
	Infected (cm.)	*Non-infected* (cm.)	*Difference* (cm.)
All neonates	47·5 (83)	48·8 (447)	+1·3
All males	47·5 (38)	49·0 (243)	+1·5
All females	47·5 (45)	48·4 (204)	+0·9

(−) Indicates number of subjects in group.

Table VII

DIFFERENCE IN MEAN HEAD CIRCUMFERENCE* BETWEEN INFECTED
AND NON-INFECTED GROUPS

	Mean head circumference		
	Infected (cm.)	*Non-infected* (cm.)	*Difference* (cm.)
All neonates	32·4 (77)	33·1 (325)	+0·7
All males	32·4 (34)	33·3 (182)	+0·9
All females	32·3 (43)	32·9 (148)	+0·7

(−) Indicates number of subjects in group.
* This measurement was made only on the last 402 consecutive
infants.

Table VIII

DIFFERENCE IN MEAN CHEST CIRCUMFERENCE* BETWEEN
INFECTED AND NON-INFECTED GROUPS

Mean chest circumference

	Infected (cm.)	Non-infected (cm.)	Difference (cm.)
All neonates	31·1 (77)	31·8 (325)	+0·7
All males	31·2 (34)	32·1 (182)	+0·9
All females	31·0 (43)	31·8 (148)	+0·8

(–) Indicates number of subjects in group.
 * This measurement was made only on the last 402 consecutive
   neonates.

Table IX

DIFFERENCE IN MID-ARM CIRCUMFERENCE BETWEEN
INFECTED AND NON-INFECTED GROUPS

Mid-arm circumference

	Infected (cm.)	Non-infected (cm.)	Difference (cm.)
All neonates	9·7 (83)	10·3 (447)	+0·6
All males	9·8 (38)	10·3 (243)	+0·5
All females	9·7 (45)	10·2 (204)	+0·5

(–) Indicates number of subjects in group.

(c) *Chest measurement*

This measure, taken at the nipple line, showed a smaller circumference among the group with infected placentae (Table VIII).

(d) *Mid-arm circumference*

The mid-arm circumference measure was smaller in infants with infected placentae (Table IX).

Table X

DIFFERENCE IN SUBCUTANEOUS TRICEPS SKINFOLD BETWEEN INFECTED AND NON-INFECTED GROUPS

	Subcutaneous triceps skinfold		
	Infected (mm.)	*Non-infected (mm.)*	*Difference (mm.)*
All neonates	4·5 (83)	4·5 (447)	—
All males	4·5 (38)	4·5 (243)	—
All females	4·5 (45)	4·6 (204)	+0·1

(–) Denotes number of subjects in each group.

(e) *Subcutaneous triceps skinfold*

This was the only anthropometric measure which remained unaffected (Table X).

(f) *Muscle circumference*

The muscle circumference measure was found to be smaller in the infants with infected placentae ($C_2 = C_1 - \pi s$; Jelliffe and Jelliffe, 1960) (Table XI).

(g) *Fat/weight ratio*

Conversely, the fat/weight ratio (mm./kg.) was higher in the infected group (Table XII).

In present paediatric practice certain anthropometric standards are often employed in order to assess whether a

Table XI

DIFFERENCE IN MEAN MUSCLE CIRCUMFERENCE BETWEEN INFECTED AND NON-INFECTED GROUPS ($C_2 = C_1 - \pi s$)

	Mean muscle circumference		
	Infected (cm.)	Non-infected (cm.)	Difference (cm.)
All neonates	8·32 (83)	8·97 (447)	+0·47
All males	8·38 (38)	8·88 (243)	+0·50
All females	8·27 (45)	8·68 (204)	+0·41

(−) Denotes number of subjects in each group.

C_1: mid-arm circumference.
C_2: muscle circumference.
πs: skinfold.

Table XII

DIFFERENCE IN MEAN FAT/WEIGHT RATIO (mm/kg.) BETWEEN INFECTED AND NON-INFECTED GROUPS

	Fat/weight ratio (mm./kg.)		
	Infected	Non-infected	Difference
All neonates	1·59 (83)	1·47 (447)	−0·12
All males	1·60 (38)	1·44 (243)	−0·16
All females	1·57 (45)	1·50 (204)	−0·07

(−) Denotes number of subjects in each group.

neonate can be termed undersized. When these norms are applied to the infants in this study a higher percentage of undersized infants are found among the group with infected placentae (Table XIII).

These results were not altered when sex, birth rank and genetic groups were considered.

Table XIII

PERCENTAGE OF UNDERSIZED NEONATES AS JUDGED BY ACCEPTED ANTHROPOMETRIC STANDARDS

Anthropometric measurements	Infected placentae		Non-infected placentae		Difference
(total no. of neonates)	No. of neonates	%	No. of neonates	%	%
Birth weight 2,500 g. or less (66)	18	19·6	48	10·0	9·6
Birth length 47 cm. or less (118)	28	33·7	90	20·1	13·6
Head circumference 33 cm. or less (199)	57	74·0	142	43·7	30·3
Chest circumference 33 cm. or less (37)	14	18·4	23	7·4	11·0
Weight/length ratio 53·2 or less (51)	12	14·5	39	8·5	6·0

Placentae

One hundred unselected placentae were weighed. Of these 13 were found to be parasitized and although no significant macroscopical differences were found, the mean weight of the infected placentae was 45·3 g. less than the weight of the parasite-free placentae.

Plasmodial infections

The dominant parasite found was *Plasmodium falciparum*, which accounted for 54·4 per cent of all infections. Smears

of placental bloods infected with this species of
Plasmodium presented a striking appearance of intense
parasitic activity. In a further 20·7 per cent of slides large
masses of phagocytized pigment were much in evidence;
20·7 per cent showed the presence of *Plasmodium malariae*
parasites and 4·3 per cent showed mixed infections of
P. falciparum and *P. malariae*.

DISCUSSION

The cause of low birth weight in developed regions has
been the focus of numerous important studies and many
factors have been incriminated.

In the present study, socioeconomic group, birth rank
and sex of neonate, and genetic variation have already
been excluded. Congenital deformities, endemic and
familial types of dwarfing, hydramnios, sickle-cell
disease, altitude and smoking during pregnancy played no
part, and there was no significant difference in range of
maternal height, weight or age in the two groups.

The beneficial effect of rest during pregnancy could also
be excluded as all these women worked in their homes and
fields until term. The presence of bacterial and viral
infections could not be ascertained, nor could bacilluria.
Nor could more esoteric tests to evaluate maternal heart
size or the presence of uterine deformities by hysterography
be performed. Only one case of placenta praevia, two cases
of pre-eclamptic toxaemia, one case of cardiac disease,
and two cases of diabetes were found in this series, and all
their infants weighed over 2,500 g.

Maternal emotional stress could not be evaluated, nor
could "maternal growth constraint" be tested, as the birth
weight of other siblings was not available (Ounsted,
1965).

The difficult problem of assessing maternal nutritional
status remained. No woman appeared severely malnourished,

and the mean weight-for-height levels of both groups fell within the "desirable" range (D. B. Jelliffe, 1966). Some of them (4·0 per cent) had poor musculature as judged clinically and 1·2 per cent could be considered obese. Fifteen women had a mild follicular keratosis, one woman showed evidence of glossitis, and two had enlarged parotids; no gross oedema of the extremities was seen and no other possible nutritional stigmata were evident. There was no difference in maternal weights, heights or incidence of these minor clinical stigmata in the two groups.

Fifty-eight per cent of the women had some conjunctival pallor, most of these (65·2 per cent) being in the group with infected placentae.

Direct questioning and food-consumption studies undertaken in the homes of women of a similar socioeconomic group have revealed (Rutishauser, 1965, personal communication) that the daily protein intake, mainly derived from vegetable sources, varied from 34 g. to 75 g. (calorific values 1,704 to 2,590). It is felt that the women in the present study would make no additional allowance for the physiological needs of pregnancy and possibly food taboos would further restrict protein intake of eggs, fish and certain meats could they have been financially afforded.

If seasonal variations were considered, it could be postulated that "wet season" babies would be smaller, due to the increased numbers of anopheline mosquitoes present, a higher incidence of infected placentae and a possible poorer maternal dietary owing to the seasonal food shortage at the beginning of the rains.

CONCLUSIONS

Any factors which impede a reliable and nutritious maternal blood supply to the foetus, or affect the efficiency of the placenta as a supply organ, or interfere with actual placental foetal circulation, will tend to influence adversely the birth weight of the neonate. In the present study the mechanism of foetal growth failure remains to be elucidated, but unfortunately some vital information is lacking and the actual cause of this growth retardation cannot be clearly ascertained.

Firstly, the gestational period could not be determined and one is faced with the all-too-familiar riddle: were these babies with infected placentae "small-for-dates" or infants prematurely expelled from their uterine environment? Obstetrically, it could be argued that a severe or chronic fever could precipitate a premature delivery, but the mothers in this series appeared to be clinically well at the time of delivery.

Next, it must be stressed that the duration of the maternal infection was unknown, and possibly foetal growth would be more influenced by a longer exposure to placental malaria.

Garnham (1938-39), in his detailed work on the placenta in malaria with special reference to reticuloendothelial immunity, notes that ". . . in certain phases of malaria, the intervillous spaces which should contain nothing but blood, are an almost solid mass of reticuloendothelial cells and it is difficult to understand how the foetus is nourished. In fact, many of the abortions in malaria would appear to be due to the deaths of the foetus through a physical interference with the circulation of the placental blood, rather than the direct effect of malarial toxins." This well-known picture of schizogony and reticulo-endothelial phagocytosis which appears after the fourth month of pregnancy is associated with *P. falciparum* infections and the largest numbers of reticuloendothelial cells are found in cases of chronic malaria. Garnham further estimated that in *P. falciparum* infections over 60 per cent of the red cells could be infected.

When the metabolic needs of the malarial parasites are envisaged, it must be recalled that glucose, laevulose, maltose and glycerol are oxidized by the parasites, and riboflavin, calcium pantothenate, folic acid, biotin and oxygen are among the substances required for their metabolism; the foetus is also competing for supplies of oxygen and glucose vital for its growth.

Maegraith (1948), applying the figures of oxygen consumption of *Plasmodium cynomolgi* to the malaria of man, estimated that if 1 per cent of the red blood cells were infected, the parasites would require 2 ml. of oxygen per minute compared to the basal requirements of a whole man of probably 220 ml. per minute.

Hytten and Leitch (1964), reviewing the literature on oxygen requirements in human reproduction, concluded that the metabolic rate of the foetus would be, weight for weight, not greater than that of a resting fasting non-pregnant woman. A standard woman weighing 56 kg. would have a basal metabolic requirement of 1,400 cal. a day or 200 ml. of oxygen per minute; her foetus weighing 3·3 kg. at

term would require 12 ml. of oxygen a minute $\left(\dfrac{200 \times 3 \cdot 3}{56} \right)$

a standard placenta (700 g.) 3·7 ml./min., and the uterus 3·3 ml./min.

If it is possible to correlate these findings of parasite and host requirements for oxygen, bearing in mind the heavy parasitic load in the placenta, one can but wonder to what degree of anoxia the foetus will have been exposed and what other necessary nutrients will have been witheld from it.

Sinclair and Silverman (1966), in their studies of oxygen consumption of infants post-term (two to ten days) under resting thermoneutral conditions, used their findings as an index of intrauterine growth in "active tissue mass" and concluded that neonates who had been undergrown *in utero* consumed as a group more oxygen per kilogram body weight than did normally grown babies of a similar birth weight; this did not apply when babies of a similar gestational period were compared, although the most undergrown babies showed a tendency to be hypermetabolic even for the duration of gestation. These results may suggest that growth rate could be a better indication of oxygen and calorie requirements in neonates than birth weight alone. One could speculate once more against what odds the babies with infected placentae were struggling to receive oxygenation from a placenta becoming deficient in this necessary substance.

It is possible that studies on oxygen saturation in the umbilical vein of babies with infected placentae might prove of interest. Minkowski (1959) concluded in his studies on newborns that a 50 per cent oxygen saturation level in the umbilical vein was the critical one below which serious neurological anomalies occurred. A follow-up study, when practicable, of infants with an infected placenta and a subnormal head circumference could prove valuable in assessing possible brain damage, if a relative anoxia occurs in these cases.

The lighter the neonate the more expensive per ounce a commodity he becomes, when one considers the prolonged and costly neonatal hospitalization period and possible future readmittances. If these infants survive one could dispassionately ponder on the usefulness to the community of these possibly brain-damaged new citizens.

In developing areas with either indifferent acceptability or poor facilities for family planning, where these babies of low birth weight are a recurring problem, it would seem imperative that preventive measures be instituted and the logical step to take would seem to be the distribution of anti-malarial drugs at prenatal clinics.

No teratogenic effects of chloroquine on the foetus appear to occur when it is given in the dosages required to prevent malaria. Morley, Woodland and Cuthbertson (1964), who gave weekly doses of pyrimethamine to a group of pregnant women living in a malarious region of Nigeria and a placebo to a control group of mothers, reported that babies born of mothers who had received anti-malarials were 187 g. heavier than those born to the non-treated group. Colbourne (1955) demonstrated that the distribution of anti-malarial drugs did not appear to cause undue interference with malarial immunity in indigenous African populations.

Despite the problem which cephalo-pelvic disproportion poses in many African communities most tropical obstetricians would appear to agree that anti-malarial drugs would prove beneficial.

With these encouraging results, if the initial financial outlay for the distribution of anti-malarial drugs is made possible by government agencies, this measure apart from its humanitarian aspects and its economy in future financial commitments could prove a realistic link in the chain of endeavours to improve maternal and child health services in developing countries.

SUMMARY

Placental malaria and foetal growth failure

A study was undertaken among parturient African women in Kampala, Uganda, to evaluate the incidence of placental malaria and to assess its effect on foetal growth. Five hundred and seventy women and their live-born singleton neonates and placentae were examined; $16 \cdot 1$ per cent of the women had placental malarial infection.

The birth weight of neonates born with an infected placenta was 263 g. less than the weight of the non-infected babies (statistically highly significant: $P = <0 \cdot 001$), and this remained unaffected when birth rank, sex of neonate and tribe were considered.

All other anthropometric measurements—length, head chest, mid-arm and muscle circumferences—were similarly affected, but there was no variation in subcutaneous skinfold values between the two groups.

Hypotheses to account for this foetal growth failure are considered, including possible effects of placental malarial parasites on foetal anoxia and nutrient supply.

The advantages and problems of distribution of anti-malarial tablets to pregnant women in endemic malarious regions are discussed.

REFERENCES

Archibald, H. M. (1956). *Bull. Wld Hlth Org.*, **15**, 842.
Archibald, H. M. (1958). *Br. med. J.*, **2**, 1562.
Bruce-Chwatt, L. J. (1952). *Ann. trop. Med. Parasit.*, **46**, 173.
Cannon, D. S. H. (1958). *Br. med.J.*, **2**, 877.
Clarke, H. C. (1915). *J. exp. Med.*,**22**, 47.
Colbourne, M. J. (1955). *Trans. R. Soc. trop. Med. Hyg.*, **49**, 5.
Garnham, P. C. C. (1938-39). *Trans. R. Soc. trop. Med. Hyg.*, **32**, 13.
Hytten, F. E., and Leitch, I. (1964). In *The Physiology of Human Pregnancy*, p. 205. Oxford: Blackwell Scientific Publications.
Jelliffe, D. B. (1966). *The Assessment of the Nutritional Status of the Community. Monograph Ser. W.H.O.*, No. 53.
Jelliffe, D. B., and Jelliffe, E. F. P. (1960). *Am. J. publ. Hlth.*, **50**, 1355.
Jelliffe, E. F. P. (1966). *J. trop. Pediat.*, **12**, Monogr. 2, p. 19..
Maegraith, B. G. (1948). *Pathological Processes in Malaria and Blackwater Fever*. Oxford: Blackwell Scientific Publications.
McLaren, D. S., and Ward, P. G. (1962). *E. Afr. med. J.*, **39**, 182.
Minkowski, A. (1959). In *Oxygen Supply to the Human Foetus*, p. 275. Oxford: Blackwell Scientific Publications.
Morley, D., Woodland, M., and Cuthbertson, W. F. J. (1964). *Br. med. J.* **1**, 667.
Ounsted, M. (1965). *Dev. Med. Child Neurol.*, **7**, 479. (Quoted in *Lancet, 1*, 587, 1966).
Rutishauser, I. (1965). Personal communication.
Sinclair, J. C., and Silverman, W. A. (1966). *Pediatrics, Springfield* **38**, 48.
Spitz, A. J. W. (1959). *Bull. Wld Hlth Org.*, **21**, 242.

Acknowledgement

This study was made possible by a research grant from the World Health Organization.

DISCUSSION

Maegraith: It is nice to have a piece of work which has been so carefully controlled in such difficult circumstances. People who live in sophisticated countries seldom realize the difficulties of tackling such a problem in the field.

I should like to disagree to some extent with Maegraith (1948, *loc. cit.*). We have come a long way since then. We have studied this question of the competition between the parasite and the host animal but we haven't done any work on babies or infants. It has become quite clear that it is only the more extreme examples of infection that have any direct importance in the metabolism of the host.

When we talk about anoxia we must distinguish between the two main groups: anoxic anoxia, which is a genuine deficiency of oxygen, and cytotoxic anoxia, in which there may be enough oxygen but the cell is unable to use it because of some metabolic disturbance.

It is interesting that as *P. falciparum* or *P. knowlesi* infections develop in monkeys and glyconeogenesis ceases in the liver, sugar metabolism can to some extent be restored by adrenal extracts such as cortisone. We have now also been able to identify a factor in human serum in falciparum malaria, and in monkey and mouse malaria, which knocks out the oxidative phosphorylation and respiration of active mitochondria. As this is a soluble substance, interchange at the placenta might have an effect on the infant. For 20-odd years I have talked against the existence of malaria toxins, but now I think I must support it.

Mrs. Jelliffe, in the child who had parasites in the blood at birth, was there any placental damage?

Mrs. Jelliffe: Yes; this child was delivered by Caesarian section after a long labour, and the placenta was extremely ragged and rather dark in colour. In another case I found some *P. falciparum* parasites in the cord, but despite examination of 500 fields of neonatal blood I found no parasites.

Hendrickse: Have you any further data on maternal haemoglobin values?

Mrs. Jelliffe: No, I am afraid this was not possible. I just looked at the conjunctival pallor, which I realise is most inadequate.

Hendrickse: In our hospital we now have a lot of evidence to show that malaria in pregnancy tends to precipitate megaloblastic anaemia due to folic acid deficiency. If malaria is controlled during pregnancy by the use of pyrimethamine (which is itself a folic acid antagonist) the incidence of megaloblastic anaemia is reduced. Folic acid deficiency would thus seem to be one of the factors which might be responsible for, or at least contribute to, the low birth weight of babies born to women with malaria in pregnancy.

Maegraith: I was surprised to hear that the sickle-cell trait appeared to have no effect on parasites in the placenta in malaria. My recollection is that some workers in Ghana had found that the distribution was much as would have been expected, and that the same applies to glucose-6-phosphate dehydrogenase deficiency (unpublished data).

Mrs. Jelliffe: No woman was suffering from sickle-cell anaemia. I haven't had the sickle-cell trait results statistically analysed yet, but there did not appear to be much difference in incidence of the sickle-cell trait in mothers with non-infected (14·8 per cent) and those with infected placentae (13·0 per cent).

Morley: We were fortunate in having Dr. Bruce-Chwatt in Nigeria at the inception of our study to advise us on our course of action. The mothers were given two tablets of pyrimethamine once a month, for four months, the cost of the tablets being approximately 8d. per pregnancy; in addition they received chloroquin if they attended with fever. The total cost would be small if this treatment proved to be suitable on a wide scale.

An unexpected finding was that mothers on pyrimethamine gained more weight during their pregnancy. The group on pyrimethamine showed an increase in weight of 1 lb. 14 oz. (0·85 kg.) compared with the control group on lactose. Since the average gain was only 6 lb. (3·6 kg.) this was 23 per cent of the gain in weight and this is further evidence of the advantageous effect of avoiding malaria in pregnancy.

In Nigeria primiparous mothers have something like a 37 per cent chance of having an infected placenta, whereas at a parity of 7 they have only a 14 per cent chance (Morley, D., Woodland, M., and Cuthbertson, W. J. F. [1964]. *Br. med. J.*, 2, 667-668). This would suggest that the mother herself in subsequent pregnancies has increased her resistance to malaria.

Berry: If the skinfold measurement was equal in the infected and uninfected babies, can it be deduced that the caloric supply was equally adequate in the two?

Mrs. Jelliffe: I feel I cannot necessarily make this assumption.

Maegraith: What has been your experience with congenital infection?

Mrs. Jelliffe: This is the first time I have found parasites in the blood of an infant examined immediately after birth.

Brock: Are you defining congenital malaria as the recovery of parasites in the newborn child?

Mrs. Jelliffe: Yes, on the day of birth in live babies. I did not
examine the blood of any stillborn infants with placental malaria
in this study, as they had already been removed from the
delivery room. Records of autopsies at Mulago Hospital in Kampala
(1953-64) showed the presence of malarial pigment in the liver
and spleen of only one out of 99 babies born alive but dying
subsequently on the day of birth. Dr. G. Wickramasurya (1953.
J. Obstet. Gynaec. Br. Emp., 42, 816) in Ceylon found parasites
in the brain and in other tissues of five stillborn infants, during
a malaria epidemic, and Sir Gordon Covell (1950. *Trop. Dis. Bull.*,
47, 1147) has reviewed the literature on 107 cases of congenital
malaria (infants delivered full term, prematurely or stillborn)
from different areas of the world.

Brock: Are these not cases of so-called malarial abortion?

Mrs. Jelliffe: It has been stated that malaria is responsible for
abortions, though it is difficult to prove this. I examined blood
taken from 118 aborted placentae and 15 per cent of them showed
the presence of malarial parasites. Ringform parasites are not
often seen before the fourth month of pregnancy, and these were
all more mature placentae.

Maegraith: It is difficult to understand how the infection can
get through in the absence of an injury to the placenta. From all
that we know about the parasites at the moment I am satisfied at
any rate that the merozoites which come from the blood (E) forms
do not penetrate back into the tissues. I would have been very
happy if you had been able to show that this was the case.

Mrs. Jelliffe: Apart from malaria, microfilariae were seen in 4
per cent of all placentae examined, and also in two cord bloods,
but I found none in neonatal bloods. In the products of one
evacuation, I found a great many microfilariae, and it is possible
that this infection might have caused a miscarriage.

Vahlquist: In healthy pregnant women signs of direct contact
between the mother's blood and the foetal blood are not infrequently
found. For instance, the offspring of healthy mothers may have
antibodies to *E. coli* of O type, which are normally not passed on
and which could only be explained by small ruptures. It is
surprising that these placentae which you have described so well
and which are grossly changed pathologically do not very often
show extensive anatomical changes, with ruptures. If parasites
are passed on to the foetus could it be that newborn babies have
differing susceptibilities to malaria?

Maegraith: I shall be discussing that in my paper.

Jelliffe: One of the present interests in paediatric nutrition is
the interdependence of the mother and child, and the placenta is
of obvious importance. This is particularly so in tropical

paediatrics, because it is so imperative to ensure that the
newborn baby has the maximum stores of all possible nutrients.

The question of malarial impact on the mother during pregnancy, on the foetus and on the newborn child is important from
several points of view. Placental malaria introduces an
additional complication into the already very complex evaluation
of factors limiting mental development, which is also one of the
major problems at the moment in the nutritional world. From what
we have heard, the question of anoxia during the latter part of
foetal life, as produced perhaps by the malarial parasite, may
have to be taken into account, especially as the present view is
that the period of main risk of damage to the brain is probably
at −3 to +6 months.

Brock: Are you satisfied that the infected and non-infected
women had similar environmental histories, Mrs. Jelliffe?

Mrs. Jelliffe: These were all poor African women living near
Kampala. The husbands were either labourers or small peasant
farmers, but the financial differences between these two groups
were not very great; maybe during the season when the crops
were gathered the farmers would have some slight advantage.
There were no wives of government officials in this group.

Hendrickse: What is the incidence of *P. malariae* infections of
the placenta?

Mrs. Jelliffe: We found quite a lot in Uganda. In the present
study 20·7 per cent of the placentae were infected with quartan
parasites and a further 4·3 per cent showed mixed infections with
P. falciparum and *P. malariae*, with *P. falciparum* predominating.

Hendrickse: Didn't you find mainly falciparum malaria in West
Africa, Dr. Morley?

Morley: Cannon had some data on this (1958. *Br. med. J.*, 2,
877). These children were mostly delivered in villages and it was
not easy to get hold of the placentae.

Mrs. Jelliffe: From the cases of placental malaria in which the
species was identified *P. falciparum* would appear to dominate
the West African scene, though Bruce-Chwatt (1952, *loc. cit.*)
reported mixed *P. falciparum* and *P. malariae* in 0·6 per cent
of placentae. In East Africa, McLaren and Ward (1952, *loc. cit.*)
found *P. vivax* in some placentae and Garnham (1935, *loc. cit.*)
reported a few cases of *P. malariae.* All three species were
mentioned as infecting the placenta in Covell's review (1950)
of congenital malaria.

Brock: It is usually said that falciparum malaria accounts for
90 per cent of the malaria throughout the African continent, yet
you found a considerably lower percentage.

Mrs. Jelliffe: In the present study *P. falciparum* predominated
(54·4 per cent of all infections). In a further 20·7 per cent of

placentae large masses of phagocytized pigment were seen, suggesting a recent massive infection with *P. falciparum*. However, the incidence of *P. malariae* may be on the increase in Uganda (Jelliffe, E. F. P. [1967]. *Trop. geogr. Med.*, **19**, 15). D. F. Clyde has reported an apparent rise in quartan malaria in the Rift Valley in Tanganyika (1965. *E. Afr. med. J.*, **39**, 528). Maybe with the more frequent use of blood transfusions we are propagating this species (Sergiev, P. G., Tiburskaya, N. R., and Vruleuskaia, O. I., quoted by Bruce-Chwatt, L. J. [1963]. *W. Afr. med. J.*, **12**, 141; Lupasco, G., *et al.*, quoted by Bruce-Chwatt, [1963], *loc. cit.*), or it may be that whereas cases with *P. falciparum* presenting with fever and detectable parasitaemia are treated, the relatively asymptomless quartan species are less likely to receive therapy and will therefore continue to persist.

Maegraith: The prevalence of *P. malariae* usually varies with the age of the patient. In West Africa *P. malariae* is very common in young children up to about the age of puberty, after which its incidence seems to drop off. There is plenty of *P. falciparum* as well, but this predominates as the *P. malariae* goes down and the age group goes up. There is some indication now that quartan malaria is spreading over a larger age group.

INTERACTION OF NUTRITION AND INFECTION

B. G. MAEGRAITH

*Department of Tropical Medicine, Liverpool School
of Tropical Medicine, Liverpool*

The introduction to the Report of the World Health
Organization Expert Committee on Nutrition and Infection
states (Expert Committee, 1965):

"The concept that malnutrition could make man more susceptible to infectious disease and also alter the course and
outcome of the resulting illness has long been current in
the history of medicine and public health. Circumstantial
evidence is plentiful, principally based on clinical experience.
Well-controlled observations have been few, and hence clear
proof in support of the concept has been slow to accumulate.
It has been much easier to demonstrate that infection is
often directly responsible for lowering the state of nutrition.

The fact that infectious diseases were widespread in the
same regions of the world as those in which malnutrition
also prevailed led gradually to a realization that the two
phenomena might be inter-related."

Later in the same WHO Report an interesting summary is
given of some of the major areas in which research on the
inter-reaction of infection and nutrition might be mounted.
These are: the effects of infection on nutritional status,
the effects of malnutrition on resistance to infection, and
the mechanisms involved in the interaction, including the
possibility that in some instances abnormal nutrition or
malnutrition may lead to changes in the infectious agent
itself. These suggestions are worth consideration, since
the interactions of nutrition and infection are clearly basic
factors in the parasite : host and host : parasite relationships. The surprising fact that relatively little is known

41

about the problem probably arises largely from difficulties encountered in coming to grips with it.

Apart from the intrinsic problem of obtaining reliable statistics, in such a complex interplay of biological processes it is not easy to plan or execute controlled trials or experiments either in clinical medicine or in academic research. On the whole, it has proved easier to define the effects of infection on host nutrition rather than the reverse. Nevertheless, there is evidence which indicates that the nutritional status of the host may have profound effects on the progress of certain infectious agents. Progress in this respect may be modified in either direction. So far as the incidence of human malaria is concerned, there is some indication that incidence is high where the population is badly nourished, but there is little to support the generally accepted view that this also applies to the severity of individual infections and resulting mortality. Indeed, there is some evidence that the most serious effects of *Plasmodium falciparum* infection may be mollified in malnourished (as compared with well-fed) children.

Thus Edington (1967) has claimed that cerebral malaria is rarely seen in children suffering from kwashiorkor and both Gilles and Hendrickse (personal communications) have noted that death from *P. falciparum* occurs more often in well-nourished than badly nourished children. On the other hand, malaria is commonly regarded as one of the greatest contributors to mortality and morbidity in the age group 0 to 5 years in holo-endemic and highly endemic areas.

In the experimental field the nutritional situation in the host is demonstrably important in malaria. I refer here only to mammalian malaria. There is ample information indicating that the parasite may be influenced by the host diet in avian malaria but the results are difficult to interpret and are not necessarily relevant to mammalian malaria, since the avian erythrocyte is nucleated.

Deficiency of ascorbic acid prolongs the course of *Plasmodium knowlesi* infection. *Plasmodium berghei* malaria in rats is depressed by starvation, by a ketogenic diet and by pyridoxine deficiency; the infection is suppressed in mice given a diet rich in cod liver oil, a situation which is reversible by the addition of vitamin E.

Malaria and the host diet

A most interesting observation in this respect was our own demonstration that *P. berghei* infection in rats could be completely suppressed by placing the animals on a milk diet (Maegraith, Deegan and Jones, 1952). The addition of para-aminobenzoic acid (PABA) to the milk diet partly restored the activity of the parasites (Hawking, 1953).

Bray and Garnham (1953) subsequently showed that a milk diet similarly suppressed sporozite-induced *Plasmodium cynomolgi* malaria in monkeys; we confirmed this in animals given human milk. We subsequently found that blood-transmitted *P. knowlesi* infection was equally well suppressed when *Macaca mulatta* was placed on a milk diet. Later a human experiment with sporozoite-induced *Plasmodium vivax* malaria was carried out. The results (unpublished) were vitiated by circumstances outside our control, but they clearly indicated similar suppression of the infection in volunteers on a milk diet.

The suppression of malaria parasites in a host on a milk diet naturally led us to suggest that herein might lie the explanation of the common observation that severe *P. falciparum* malaria is rarely seen in very young infants, even in highly endemic areas. The suggestion has been criticized on the grounds that in some parts of Africa mother's milk contains adequate quantities of PABA. This observation is difficult to correlate with the suppression of *P. knowlesi* in monkeys on a diet of human milk. It may be that the availability of the amino acid in the milk is an important factor.

McGregor, Gilles and Fuller (1956) examined *P. falciparum* infections in 105 infants in the Gambia and found that five of 18 infants (exclusively on breast milk) in the age group 0 to 5 weeks were infected with an average parasite density of 1,220 in 200 oil-immersion fields. Thirty-three of 46 breast-fed infants and four of six infants in the age group six to 15 weeks on a diet of dried milk plus supplements were infected, the respective densities being 5,955 and 17,520. In the age group 16 to 25 weeks 14 of 14 breast-fed infants and 16 of 21 on dried milk and supplement were also infected, with parasitic densities of 4,742 and 1,769 respectively.

PABA was present in somewhat lower than normal amounts in samples of mother's milk taken on two separate occasions. McGregor, Gilles and Fuller then added PABA to the diet of a group of seven infants and a placebo of lactose to another group of seven infants over the period from birth to six months of age. Four of the first group and two of the second contracted falciparum malaria. The authors concluded that in the Gambia a diet of breast milk alone did not protect an infant from malaria infection.

This conclusion can, I think, be challenged on the grounds that in the age groups 0 to 5 weeks and six to 15 weeks there was, despite the authors' statement to the contrary, a significantly lower density of parasitaemia in the breast-fed infants than in infants given supplements. This does not obtain in the group aged 16 to 25 weeks.

The importance of considering densities of infection as well as incidence has been clearly demonstrated by Allison (1954) and subsequent workers who studied the protective effect of haemoglobin S against *P. falciparum* malaria and more recently the protective activity of glucose-6-phosphate dehydrogenase (G-6-PD) in *P. falciparum* infection.

Kretschmar (1966) has now provided evidence based on the densities of infection in infants in Nigeria which supports our original contention. This author studied a group of children in Western Nigeria infected with *P. falciparum* and compared densities of infection in infant age groups with diets which were classified as follows: mother's milk only; mother's milk and milk powder; mother's milk and other food; milk powder and other food. He found that densities of infection were low on the all-milk diets and increased as the milk content of the diet was reduced. He concluded that the resistance of suckling children to *P. falciparum* malaria was clearly associated with their diet, i.e. with the ingestion of milk.

The importance of studying density of infection is obvious, in view of the experimental work on animals quoted above, since there is apparently no evidence of prevention of infection during a milk diet. We reported suppression of infection and in our animals the parasites became overt when the normal diet was restored.

Other workers, including Kretschmar, have observed that during suppression of infection in a host placed on various diets (all-milk or all-meat) immunogenic processes may continue. In this way, resistance to infection can be built up, as was demonstrated by Adler and Gunders (1965), who protected susceptible mice against a virulent strain of *Plasmodium vinckei* by keeping them on an all-meat diet before infection and subsequently for 10 to 14 days. On their return to a normal diet most animals survived and subsequently resisted further challenge by the parasite, which normally killed 100 per cent of infected animals. This is a nice example of the importance of host nutrition in resisting the development and toxic effects of a parasite without apparently interfering with its immunogenic properties. In a way it almost amounts to using the suppressed parasite as a vaccine. Studies in this field might well be important eventually in human malaria.

Other parasites and host diet

Other parasites as well as plasmodia have been found to be sensitive to the diet of the host. There is evidence, for instance, that the multiplication of *Entamoeba histolytica* and sometimes its invasive powers can be influenced by host diet: a milk diet impedes its development after intra-caecal injection into guinea pigs; a diet deficient in vitamin C increases its invasiveness in the same animal; a diet of salmon meat enhances its activity in the colons of dogs.

The importance of the protein content of the diet has recently been shown in *Toxocara canis* infection in puppies (Platt and Heard, 1965). Heavy infections occurred in animals reared on a low protein diet. Infection was minimal on an adequate protein diet.

Infection and the intestinal absorption of foodstuffs

The examples mentioned above show that host nutrition can be important in the development and activity of a parasitic infection. In the situations quoted the diet of the host was deliberately changed or controlled, and the possibility that the nutritional status of the host might be changed by the infection itself was not a primary consideration. However, there is ample evidence in specific instances to show that this latter effect may be an important factor in host:parasite relationships.

It is not possible to review the literature here, but it is worth mentioning a few observations on hookworm infection. Darke (1959) has shown that heavily infected African subjects absorb significantly less nitrogen from ingested food than do uninfected individuals. Somewhat similar findings have been recorded in *Nippostrongylus muris* infections in rats. In this case the absorptive failure with reduction of nitrogen retention (most of the loss was in the urine) was noted only when the animals were living on a low protein diet. Reversible (after worming) malabsorption of foodstuffs has also been described in human patients by some authors and not detected by others. These variable results may well be explicable, as in rat hookworm, in terms of the host diet. Impairment of absorption of folic acid and vitamin B_{12} have also been demonstrated (the latter also in acute amoebic liver abscess: Devakul, Areekul and Viravan, 1967).

In Liverpool we have recently been studying the effect of infection on intestinal absorption in animals infected with malaria and hookworm, since in both infections the diet of the host has been found important in the development of the parasite or its pathogenic effects, or both (for example the milk diet quoted above in malaria, and the importance of iron reserve in the evolution of hookworm anaemia). The specific problems we have considered are—can a general infection, such as *P. knowlesi* in *M. mulatta*, and an infection localized (eventually) in the intestine, such as *Ancylostoma caninum* in dogs, influence the nutritional state of the host by affecting the absorption of foodstuffs and other substances across the intestinal membrane?

I give below the results of our experiments in some detail, since they illustrate one method of attacking the problem which should be used more widely, not only in the laboratory (as described here) but also in clinical studies. In fact, similar work in man is already in progress in the Hospital for Tropical Diseases in Bangkok. The basic experimental work on *P. knowlesi* malaria is being carried out in Liverpool by my colleague Panata Migasena and that in hookworm infection by Sricharoen Migasena, both lecturers in the School of Tropical Medicine, Bangkok. I have to thank them for allowing me to refer to the results, some of which have not yet been published.

Methods were similar in both sets of experiments involving both *P. knowlesi* and *A. caninum* infections.

The intestinal absorption curves of the following were measured in normal animals and in animals at various stages of *P. knowlesi* and *A. caninum* infections:

Xylose: Oral administration of 10 g. or 5 g. followed by biochemical assay of plasma samples.

Radioactive α-aminoisobutyric acid: 5-10 μC in 50 ml. distilled water given orally or by stomach tube followed by radioactive assay of plasma samples at intervals after ingestion.

[^{131}I]*Triolein:* After thyroid saturation with Lugol's iodine solution, the animals were given 10 μC [^{131}I]triolein in 10 ml. olive oil, 4 ml. Tween 80 and 35 ml. homogenized milk powder. Plasma (venous blood) was assayed for radioactivity at intervals after ingestion.

ABSORPTION CURVES IN *P. KNOWLESI* MALARIA AND
IN *A. CANINUM* INFECTIONS

Malaria

The infection with the Nuri strain of *P. knowlesi* caused
in *M. mulatta* a rapidly progressive fatal disease which
lasted seven to ten days from the end of the prepatent
period. Over the last three to four days the animals became
ill, and in the present series of studies all developed
"lytic" infections with terminal haemoglobinaemia and
haemoglobinuria.

Absorption curves were drawn before infection in each
animal and again in the later stages of infection when the
animal showed clinical and physical signs of the infection
and the packed cell volume (PCV) was 30 per cent or
lower.

Xylose: Changes in absorption curves could be detected
up to three days before the death of the animal. They
became more pronounced in the terminal 24 hours.

Both the absorption and plasma clearance of the sugar
were depressed. The normal absorption peak at one to two
hours after ingestion was absent and the climb to maximum
levels was slow. The plasma concentration usually
continued rising after the third hour. Since a constant
fraction is excreted, and no information is available on
altered metabolism of this sugar in the infected animals
this was taken to indicate some failure of renal excretion.

a-Aminoisobutyric acid: In infected animals the
absorption curve was depressed by the fifth day. There was
seldom a clear peak concentration and the plateau level
reached by the third hour was either maintained or the
curve rose slightly by the fifth hour.

[^{131}I]*Triolein:* The absorption curve was considerably
depressed. There was delay in reaching the maximum
plasma concentration (12 hours as compared with five in
the normal animal) and the clearance was very slow, even
after 24 hours.

Hookworm infection

Curves were drawn in dogs before infection and at various times after infection with *A. caninum*. "Acute" infections were studied less than three months after infection, "chronic" after six months.

Xylose: In acute and chronic infection (whether heavy or moderate), the changes noted were similar. The peak levels reached were lower than normal at one hour but from two hours onwards the curves followed the normal steady fall to low levels by the fifth hour.

α-Aminoisobutyric acid: Amino-acid absorption was depressed and delayed in both acute and chronic infections, more so in the chronic. Clearance was normal. The degree of infection had no significant effect.

[^{131}I]*Triolein:* In normal animals a peak of absorption was reached in one to two hours after ingestion. There followed a high plateau and later a marked fall at 12 hours, with a low plateau level persisting up to 24 hours.

Acute infections depressed the whole curve notably; there was a much lower peak absorption, occurring later than normal, and followed by a progressive fall which flattened out after 12 hours.

Chronic infection was accompanied by a curve very similar in shape to the normal absorption curve but at significantly lower levels. The plateau was reached at 12 hours at a lower level than normal but at about the same concentration as in the acute infection. The effect was less marked than in the acute infection.

THE EFFECTS OF ADRENERGIC BLOCKADE AND OF PITRESSIN (VASOPRESSIN) ON ABSORPTION IN NORMAL AND IN INFECTED ANIMALS

In order to examine the possibility that the state of the microcirculation in the intestinal wall might have some influence on absorption of amino acid and xylose, studies were made in both normal and infected animals using

phenoxybenzamine (adrenergic blocking agent), injected
intravenously one hour before the relevant absorption test,
and the hormone Pitressin, given intravenously one hour
before or intramuscularly 15 minutes before the test.

NORMAL ANIMALS

Xylose: Phenoxybenzamine had no apparent effect.
Pitressin, on the other hand, caused delay in absorption,
with lower than normal maximum values and some delay in
clearance.

a-Aminoisbutyric acid: Phenoxybenzamine administration
was followed by a very high peak occurring in the first
hour, and then by a normal clearance curve.

Pitressin greatly delayed absorption in the normal animal,
and this was followed by a rise to a plateau level which
was maintained at the fifth hour.

INFECTED ANIMALS

Malaria

Xylose: Phenoxybenzamine restored the absorption curve
of xylose to approximately normal shape, with normal peak
concentration occurring at the normal time of one to two
hours. The plasma clearance (which was delayed by the
infection) also approximated to normal.

a-Aminoisobutyric acid: Phenoxybenzamine restored the
absorption curve to normal shape, with a somewhat reduced
peak concentration, provided it was given at least one hour
before the absorption test was conducted. Given only ten
minutes before it had no effect.

Hookworm infection

Xylose : Neither phenoxybenzamine nor Pitressin had
any effect on the depressed absorption curves in the
infected animals.

a-Aminoisobutyric acid: Phenoxybenzamine had no effect.
Pitressin caused acute delay in absorption, with a low peak

concentration at about two hours (compared with the normal half-hour) and some delay in clearance.

DISCUSSION

Malaria

In the late stages of *P. knowlesi* malaria in rhesus monkeys, we have found that changes occur in the curves of absorption from the gut of a-aminoisobutyric acid, xylose and triolein. Thus, during the acute disease there is some intestinal dysfunction which affects the absorption of substances which can be regarded as representing the three basic foodstuffs. If continuous, such absorption failures might influence considerably the nutritional status of the host. As pointed out below, the effects of the adrenergic blocking agent and of Pitressin may be interpreted as indicating that the changes in absorption produced during the infection are related to dynamic changes in the circulation of blood through the gut mucosa and possibly through the liver.

In malaria we are thus probably dealing mainly with an acute physiological disturbance in the gut membrane, involving the microcirculation of blood and possibly also intestinal movements (not yet studied).

Hookworm infection

The changes in absorption curves noted in *A. caninum* infection in dogs, so far as xylose and the amino acid are concerned, are different from those detected during malaria. The picture is one of reduced peak absorption, representing some initial delay, although the final plateau is within normal limits. Changes in triolein absorption are similar in acute infections but are less pronounced in chronic infections.

The overall change in absorption in the hookworm infection thus seems largely to be one of degree. However,

the absence of any effect of the blocking agent on the
absorption curves indicates basic differences between the
absorptive lesions present in this infection and those in
malaria.

Studies of the anatomy of the relevant area of the gut
have shown that some degree of villous atrophy develops
during the hookworm infection. This may affect absorption,
as it does in other malabsorption states, by lowering the
absorptive surface, with an equivalent reduction in the
relevant blood flow. The cause of these changes in the gut
is obscure. The number of feeding areas of the worms can
hardly be enough to affect the gut surface as a whole,
although Sricharoen Migasena (1967, personal communication) has demonstrated that the areas of attachment of the
worms may reach into the wall beyond the muscularis
mucosae. It is possible that some biochemical factor is
involved.

The microcirculation in the intestinal wall

The rapid and stimulating effects of phenoxybenzamine
on the normal absorption of xylose and the amino acid
indicate not only improved absorption but also better
removal and transport elsewhere of the absorbed substances,
both of which are taken into the blood. Such an effect
could result from some relaxation of local vascular tone in
the small vessels of the intestinal mucosa. The severe
impedance of absorption caused by Pitressin, on the other
hand, could be explained partly in terms of restricted
removal resulting from the intense local vasoconstriction
invoked.

These experiments indicate that the intestinal microcirculation is actively concerned in absorption. It seems
to me that this circulation has not received the attention it
merits and I hope much more work will be done to examine
its importance in intestinal absorption in normal and
infected animals.

The reversal in *P. knowlesi* malaria of the suppressed
absorption curves for xylose and for the amino acid by

phenoxybenzamine can also be interpreted as resulting from the release of vasoconstriction in the small vessels of the absorbing mucosa. Under the circumstances this in itself might not immediately affect the absorption curves in the late stages of the infection, since it has been repeatedly demonstrated that there is a concurrent terminal portal venous vasoconstriction which is associated with a retardation of blood flow through the liver lobules (Skirrow, Chongsuphajaisiddhi and Maegraith, 1964). Such impedance of flow through the liver would clearly limit the flow from the gut.

The effect of the blocking agent on the absorption curves is uniformly demonstrable an hour after its administration. Since it has been established that the portal venous vasoconstriction is reversible by phenoxybenzamine there is a possibility that the release of intra-hepatic flows may itself have had an effect on the dependent blood flow through the gut, leading to the recorded improvement in absorption. This is supported by the absence of an effect when the blocking agent is given only ten minutes before the administration of the test substance. In this period the liver vasoconstriction has been shown to be released. Hence this release in itself has no immediate effect on absorption.

It should be noted that the blocking agent improves absorption from the normal gut, presumably by releasing local vascular tone, although it has no measurable effect on normal liver flow. Pitressin, which has a notable constrictor effect on the intestinal vessels, induces in uninfected animals abnormal absorption curves similar to those seen in malaria.

Thus the experimental evidence to date supports the view that the changes in absorption in acute malaria may be related to reduced or impeded blood flow through the intestinal wall, and possibly also to the state of the blood flow through the liver at the time.

Although a major factor in the delays in absorption in

hookworm infection may well be the anatomical changes described above, with the associated gross loss of absorptive surface, there is a strong possibility that there is an accompanying vascular defect, partly arising from the changes in the villi and supporting tissues and partly from the physiological responses of the local microcirculation. The latter is best seen in the action of Pitressin in delaying the absorption of the amino acid in both the normal and the infected animal.

It would appear from these results that one important factor in the suppression of absorption of the major foods in acute malaria may be dynamic vasoconstriction involving the intestinal blood vessels.

The physiological state of the epithelial cells of the intestinal mucosa may also contribute to the demonstrated malabsorptions, especially in malaria.

The state of activity of the mitochondria of the epithelial cells of the gut in the small intestine has not yet been determined. In view of the recorded impedance of respiration and oxidative phosphorylation in liver cell mitochondria in *P. knowlesi* malaria (Maegraith, 1966), and the equivalent electron microscope evidence of damage in these and the mitochondria of the renal epithelium, it seems probable that similar physiological lesions occur in the gut epithelium and might thus influence the absorption of substances which demand metabolic activity, though not necessarily influencing the absorption of those substances, such as xylose, which do not.

The investigations described above are incomplete. These and the conclusions drawn from the results have been considered at this stage solely to provide further discussion and to stimulate wider studies at both clinical and laboratory level.

I think the role of the gut circulation, intestinal motility, and sphincter activity in intestinal absorption in normal and infected man and other animals should be more profoundly

studied, in parallel with investigation of the disturbances that occur in general bacterial and parasitic infections and in local infections involving primarily the intestine.
Quite apart from the influence these factors may have on host nutrition and host : parasite reactions, they may well throw some light on the origin of the anorexia and nausea which are so characteristic of many infections.

Clinical studies on these lines are now being mounted, jointly in Liverpool and in the School of Tropical Medicine in Bangkok, in patients of all age groups admitted to hospital. An outline of these studies has been given here, and I hope similar patterns of research may develop elsewhere.

REFERENCES

Alder, S., and Gunders, A. E. (1965). *Israel J. med. Sci.*, **1**, 441.
Allison, A. C. (1954). *Br. med. J.*, **1**, 290.
Bray, R. S., and Garnham, P. C. C. (1953). *Br. med. J.*, **1**, 1200.
Darke, S. J. (1959). *Br. J. Nutr.*, **13**, 278.
Devakul, K., Areekul, S., and Viravan, C. (1967). *Ann. trop. Med. Parasit.*, **61**, 29.
Edington, G. (1967). Personal communication.
Expert Committee. (1965). *Nutrition and Infection. Tech. Rep. Ser. Wld Hlth Org.*, No. 314.
Hawking, F. (1953). *Br. med. J.*, **1**, 1201.
Kretschmar, W. (1966). *Fortschr. Med.*, **84**, 197.
McGregor, I. A., Gilles, H. M., and Fuller, A. T., (1956). *III Inter-African Conference on Nutrition*, Vol. 1, pp. 297-301, Luanda.
Maegraith, B. G. (1966). In *The Pathology of Parasitic Diseases*, pp. 15-32, ed. Taylor, A. E. R. Oxford: Blackwell.
Maegraith, B. G., Deegan, T., and Jones, E. S. (1952). *Br. med. J.*, **2**, 1382.
Platt, B. S., and Heard, C. R. C. (1965). *Trans. R. Soc. trop. Med. Hyg.*, **59**, 571.
Skirrow, M. B., Chongsuphajaisiddhi, T., and Maegraith, B. G. (1964). *Ann. trop. Med. Parasit.*, **58**, 502.

DISCUSSION

Brock: R. Elsdon-Dew (1945. *Nature, Lond.,* **156**, 118) and his
team in Natal have clearly shown that in Africans and Indians
living in the same villages, where hygiene is equally defective
for both groups, *Entamoeba histolytica* produces an acute serious
disease in the African but only a mild disease followed by a
carrier state in the Indian. *Entamoeba histolytica* is dependent on
a commensal bacterial flora in the gut. The striking differences
in diet between these two groups presumably produce different
environments for the *Entamoeba histolytica* within the lumen of
the intestine. Differences may also exist between the resisting
power of the mucous membrane in the two groups.

Máegraith: When I saw him recently in Liverpool, I thought
Dr. S. J. Powell sounded less confident about this Durban story.
I gathered from him that many Bantu who had moved into the
suburbs of the city got just as seriously ill with amoebic
infection as they did when they were in the bush. During the war
groups of men dropped behind the Japanese lines had to live on
what they could get locally for months on end. Though they were
all exposed to amoebic infection, relatively few became infected.
At the end of the war we estimated that something like 500,000
British troops might have returned to this country passing
Entamoeba histolytica cysts. I remember asking my chief at the
War Office what we should do about this: he thought the best
thing was not to look at their faeces. Over 20 years have elapsed
since then and very few of these men have developed active
amoebiasis.

Hendrickse: At a hospital in Durban we had contracts with
certain firms to provide medical care for their workers: one
firm housed and fed their men well, another provided housing but
no food. The difference in the nutritional state of these two
groups of urban Bantu was quite remarkable. The most severe
amoebic dysentery cases were from the poorly nourished
''bread and ginger beer group'', i.e. the group which brought their
own food which consisted largely of refined carbohydrates. When I
went to Ibadan, which has the kind of climate in which amoebic
dysentery flourishes—very poor sanitary facilities, a high
incidence of malnutrition, and so forth—it was interesting to find
that the incidence of amoebic dysentery, in adults and children,
was not nearly as bad as in Durban. In recent years the problem
of amoebic dysentery in Lagos, where there has been quite a
distinct change in living patterns, including dietary habits, has
apparently become very much worse than it is in Ibadan. This
impression is based on pathological as well as clinical evidence.

Lagos has better sanitary conditions than Ibadan, and I suspect that time will show that the increased incidence of amoebic dysentery is in some way related to changes in living habits, and in particular to changes in the diet.

Brock: In Cape Town over many years virtually the only cases of fulminant amoebiasis that we have seen have been in Africans. The interpretation of course may change but the observations seemed to me to be completely valid and well controlled.

Maegraith: I think it is Dr. Powell who is casting some doubt on the facts.

Jelliffe: Some studies done by E. C. Faust in Colombia fit in with Professor Hendrickse's remarks (Faust, E. C., and Read, T. R. [1959]. *Am. J. trop. Med. Hyg.*, 8, 293). He found that amongst the poorer section of the Colombian population *Entamoeba histolytica* occurred quite frequently in people with few or no symptoms. He also noticed that within the *Entamoeba histolytica* were starch granules derived from the poorly cooked carbohydrate foods which constituted the main diet. This suggests to me that possibly *Entamoeba histolytica* is normally a vegetarian, but that, with a diet of over-milled flour and sugar, there might be a lack of undigested starch granules in the large intestine, and it might become a carnivore!

The question Professor Gustafsson raised on the "endo-environment" of man is important. The stools of a plantain-eating Muganda, of a milk-drinking Karamojong, and of a Hadza hunter during the time of the year when he is living mostly on berries, could not be recognized with the naked eye as being the same material. These diverse diets may therefore result in endoenvironments which are as different for microflora as the human astronaut may find on Mercury, Venus and Mars.

Vahlquist: You discussed the possible influence of a milk diet on the course of malarial infection, Professor Maegraith. Have you any observations on how the diet in infants aged from 0-6 months might influence the course of malaria?

Maegraith: It might well be that the relative absence of detectable infection in early infancy might be due to the milk diet the infant is getting. McGregor, Gilles and Fuller (1956, *loc. cit.*) tried this out in Uganda and said they found nothing in it. I have recently been through their figures with Gilles and I think they fell into the same trap as we all did until Allison put us right about sickle-cell haemoglobin (Allison, A, C. [1954]. *Br. med. J.*, 1, 290). There is a big difference between the incidence of infection and the density and until Allison pointed this out no-one was quite sure about the protective value of haemoglobin S. Gilles and others (1967. *Lancet*, 1, 138) have now shown that there is something in the G-6-PD deficiency story as

well. Kretchsmar in Western Nigeria last year examined the
relation between a milk diet and parasite densities (rather than
incidence of *P. falciparum*) and showed quite clearly (1966,
loc. cit.) that there is a big difference in density values in the
child up to the age of three months living entirely on milk and the
older child who gets one addition or another to its diet. This
question should be kept wide open, because it has also been shown
that the milk of the women feeding these children is not deficient
in PABA but contains low values.

The other point to be considered is that there is some
γ-globulin present in the first two or three months of life in
African children in malarial endemic areas and it is possible that
some of this may have been passed from the mothers (Gilles, H. M.,
and McGregor, I. A. [1959]. *Ann. trop. Med. Parasit.*, **53**, 492).
Bruce-Chwatt also showed (1956. *Trans. R. Soc. trop. Med. Hyg.*,
50, 47) that in *P. berghei* infection there was some evidence in
mice that the protective γ-globulin was transmitted to the
newborn animal, but there is no evidence of this in man up to the
age of three months. Possibly both things happen but I hope
somebody will go into it again.

Garrow: Does cow's milk provide the same protection as human
milk?

Maegraith: We have tried many kinds of canned milk, goat's
milk, skimmed milk and human milk and they all had the same
effect.

HUMAN MILK AND RESISTANCE TO INFECTION*

PAUL GYÖRGY

Philadelphia General Hospital, Philadelphia, Pennsylvania

Breast-feeding reduces both morbidity and mortality rates, especially the latter. It is of special interest that infants fed human milk as compared with those fed cow's milk demonstrate higher resistance not only to intestinal disorders but also to respiratory diseases. Those like myself, whose paediatric practice dates back many decades into the pre-antibiotic era, will have no hesitation in testifying in favour of breast feeding in the prevention of infectious diseases and as the best therapeutic diet—at that time—for infants and young children with chronic and often severe acute pyogenic, especially staphylococcal, infections. Similar observations were made in chronic intestinal disorders or severe malnutrition combined with chronic infection. In general, this effect of human milk in a variety of infections was ascribed not so much to the presence of specific antibodies as to the action of unspecific factors of unknown origin. In breast-fed infants polio virus might be attacked in the intestinal tract by specific polio antibodies present in human colostrum and milk (Hodes, Berger and Hevizy, 1962; Athreya, Coriell and Charney, 1964). Transfer of immune bodies from ingested human milk through the intestine into the blood is a negligible factor in resistance to disease, if it occurs at all.

Improved general hygiene and the use of antimicrobial agents have, in more recent years, obscured the superiority

---

*Dr. György was prevented by illness from attending the meeting. The discussion is based on the precirculated abstract of his paper.

of human milk over cow's milk in regard to the figures for morbidity and mortality. However, statistical studies from countries such as the United Kingdom (Table I; Robinson, 1951) and Sweden (Table II; Sydow and Faxen, 1954; see also Mellander, Vahlquist and Mellbin, 1959), which are by no means underdeveloped, indicate that these differences may be demonstrated not only under poor but also under good hygienic conditions.

Table I

RELATION BETWEEN FEEDING AND MORTALITY AND MORBIDITY
(from Robinson, 1951)

Feeding	No. of Infants	Mortality (per 1,000)	Morbidity (per 1,000)	Case mortality (%)
Breast-fed	971	10·2	223·4	4·6
Partly bottle-fed	1441	25·7	464·2	5·5
Bottle-fed	854	57·3	573·7	10·0
Total	3266	29·3	421·3	6·9

In trying to relate resistance of the breast-fed infants to intestinal infection one has to bear in mind the nature of the intestinal flora in infants fed human milk compared with that found in artificially-fed infants. In contrast to the acid reaction of the faeces of normal breast-fed infants, the pH of the faeces of infants given the usual cow's milk formulae falls into the neutral or alkaline range. Unlike the mixed intestinal flora of infants on cow's milk formulae, the intestinal flora of healthy breast-fed infants is characterized by the prevalence of a particular species of lactobacillus, namely *Lactobacillus bifidus*.

The acid faecal reaction, together with the antibacterial fermentation products, i.e. lactate and—even more—acetate and formate, may help to suppress pathogenic or otherwise harmful intestinal bacteria, such as coliform and other proteolytic putrefying micro-organisms.

Table II

THE EFFECT OF BREAST MILK AND ARTIFICIAL FOOD ON THE INCIDENCE OF INFECTIONS IN INFANTS
0-9 MONTHS OF AGE
(from Sydow and Faxen, 1954)

Age groups, months (3-month periods)	0 - 2	1 - 3	2 - 4	3 - 5	4 - 6	5 - 7	6 - 8	7 - 9
Breast milk								
Total days of observation	1,377	1,709	1,578	1,248	923	665	430	235
Days with fever 38·1°C and above	3	5	6	8	7	6	2	4
Days with subfebrile temperature 37·6°-38·0°	26	45	59	86	85	66	23	4
Total days with rise in temperature to 37·6° and above	29	50	65	94	92	72	25	8
Artificial food								
Total days of observation	1,151	1,664	1,853	1,771	1,547	1,219	952	630
Days with fever 38·1° and above	1	10	12	20	29	34	37	24
Days with subfebrile temperature 38·6°-38·0°	52	99	146	158	165	129	94	45
Total days with rise in temperature to 37·6° and above	53	109	158	178	194	163	131	69

The growth of *Lactobacillus bifidus* in normal breast-fed infants is stimulated by the high ratio of lactose to protein and the presence of a specific bifidus growth factor in human milk (György, 1953). Chemically, the bifidus factor belongs to the group of nitrogen-containing carbohydrates. In human milk, the presence of a great variety of such neutral or acidic oligosaccharides and polysaccharides has been demonstrated. Cow's milk contains only 1/40th to 1/50th of the amount of such nitrogen-containing carbohydrates found in human milk (György, 1958).

In this connexion, reference should be made to the very interesting but not very well-known disease entity named acrodermatitis enteropathica. The disease is characterized by severe skin lesions and chronic diarrhoea, with progressive weight loss. The disease usually appears after weaning and without treatment is likely to be fatal. Brandt in 1936 stated that ". . . among all therapeutic experiments that have been initiated, the treatment with mother's milk is the only one that has any demonstrable effect . . . ". More recently, the intestinal antiseptic Diodoquin has proved to be a very effective remedy in the treatment of acrodermatitis enteropathica (Dillaha and Lorincz, 1953).

The nature of this intriguing condition is unknown; it is probably based on an inborn metabolic error, specifically on the inability of the organism to detoxify bacterial metabolites absorbed from the lumen of the intestine. Such toxic metabolites are either not formed in the intestine of breast-fed infants or are below the toxic threshold.

In the old clinical observations on the treatment of severe staphylococcal infection with (sterilized!) human milk, improvement became noticeable, not immediately as nowadays with most antibacterial agents, but after an initial period of seven to 14 days. It appeared to be a

Fig. 1. Effect of prior subcutaneous injection, for seven to 14 consecutive days, of milk and staphylococci on the survival of mice receiving a lethal dose of staphylococci. The day of challenge with the lethal dose is shown along the abscissa.

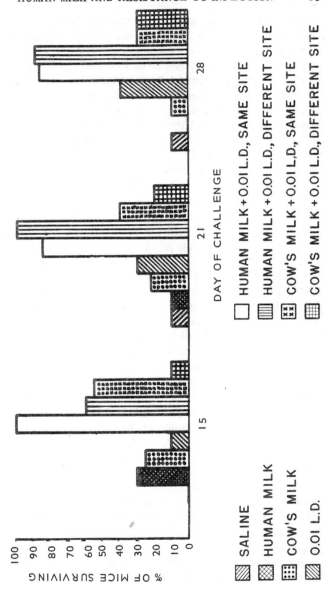

rational experimental approach to simulate these conditions in groups of mice (ten animals in each group) by injecting different groups subcutaneously, daily for seven to 14 days, with saline, human milk (0·3 ml. ≡ 30 mg.), cow's milk (0·3 ml.), 0·01 LD_{100} of fresh live staphylococci (phage type 44A), human milk (0·3 ml.) + 0·01 LD_{100} of staphylococci, cow's milk (0·3 ml.) + 0·01 LD_{100} of staphylococci. On the 15th day (or later) after the start of the initial treatment, LD_{100} of fresh staphylococci was injected intraperitoneally into all groups of mice (György, Dhanamitta and Steers, 1962).

The results clearly indicate (Fig. 1) that human milk given subcutaneously in combination with sublethal doses of virulent staphylococci is effective in giving mice significant protection against a challenge with a lethal dose of the same staphylococci. No protection was observed within the first days of the experiment and none was observed when saline or human milk was given alone. Cow's milk given alone or in combination with sublethal doses of virulent staphylococci was found to be inactive or only very weakly active. The protection of the combined pretreatment with 0·01 LD_{100} staphylococci and human milk lasted more than 14 days after termination of the initial injections. The pretreatment was in many instances also effective when the human milk and a sublethal dose (0·01 LD_{100}) of staphylococci were injected at different sites. These findings seem to indicate that the effect of human milk is not that of an adjuvant and is different from the protection given by lipopolysaccharides (Springer et al., 1961). It is probably based on some other immunological reaction, possibly on enhancement of specific antibody production.

During the past years studies have been concentrated on the fractionation and purification of the active principle in human milk involved in the increased resistance of staphylococcal infection.

The active substance (or substances) has been found to be non-dialysable and thermostable, and it is not precipitated by up to 90 per cent ethanol. The neutral fat layer of human milk was free or contained (irregularly) only traces of the principle. At high speed centrifugation (45,000 to 105,000 g) several layers are formed. The second layer is white and highly active in doses down to 0·3 or even 0·1 mg. This is tantamount to a concentration of 100 to 300-fold compared with the activity of crude human milk (30 mg.). Light petroleum in the 90 per cent alcohol filtrate produced a creamy precipitate active in doses of 0·1 mg. to 0·03 mg. Ultramicrolipograms performed in co-operation with F. Zilliken and H. Egge (Biochemisches Institut, University of Marburg, Germany) by thin-layer chromatography (unpublished experiments) make it probable that the active components, or one of them, may reside in the free fatty acid fraction. The active substance appears to be volatile and oxidizable.

Fractional molecular distillation experiments coupled with preparative gas chromatography are in progress to elucidate the fine structure of the biologically active principle.

SUMMARY

A positive effect in resistance to disease may be demonstrated in breast-fed infants (a) in gastrointestinal and (b) in parenteral infection. For gastrointestinal infection of breast-fed infants the normal acidic bacterial flora in the lower part of the intestinal tract, composed mainly of *Lactobacillus bifidus*, acts as a regulator. Low pH and the presence of fermentation products, such as lactate and especially acetate and formate, prevent the propagation of many intestinal pathogens. In parenteral infection, animal experiments demonstrated that human milk contains specific lipid constituents which appear to enhance the development of immunological defensive humoral reactions.

REFERENCES

Athreya, B. H., Coriell, L. L., and Charney, J. (1964). *J. Pediat.*, 64, 79-82.

Brandt, T. (1936). *Acta derm. vener.*, 17, 513-546.

Dillaha, C. J., and Lorincz, A. T. (1953). *Archs Derm. Syph.*, 67, 324-326.

György, P. (1953). *Pediatrics, Springfield,* 11, 98-100.

György, P. (1958). *Ciba Fdn Symp. Chemistry and Biology of Mucopolysaccharides*, pp. 140-154. London: Churchill.

György, P., Dhanamitta, S., and Steers, E. (1962). *Science,* 137, 338-340.

Hodes, H. L., Berger, R., and Hevizy, M. (1962). *Am. J. Dis. Child.*, 104, 457-459. (abstract).

Mellander, O., Vahlquist, B., and Mellbin, T. (1959). *Acta paediat., Stockh.,* 48, Suppl. 116, 11-108.

Robinson, M. (1951). *Lancet,* 1, 788-794.

Springer, G. F., Dhanamitta, S., Steers, E., Stinnett, J., and György, P. (1961). *Science,* 134, 335-336.

Sydow, G. V., and Faxen, N. (1954). *Acta paediat., Stockh.,* 43, 362-367.

DISCUSSION

[As indicated earlier, only a short abstract of Dr. György's paper was available at the time of the meeting, and some points in the following discussion would not have arisen if the full text could have been presented.—EDs.]

Aykroyd: People concerned with child health in the developing countries have the strong impression that breast feeding protects the child to a considerable extent against gastroenteritis. The infant fed mainly by the breast is less exposed to infective organisms than the infant weaned at an early stage and given diluted preparations of cow's milk out of dirty feeding bottles. Professor Jelliffe has written a great deal on this subject; I think he would like to prohibit entirely the use of feeding bottles in certain countries. These facts or impressions fit in with the idea that increasing urbanization in the developing countries is leading to an increase either in total cases of marasmus or in its prevalence relative to that of kwashiorkor. In this connexion

Professor György's observation that breast milk contains some protective substance, or substances, which guards the child against infection may be of importance.

However, I believe that in certain circumstances breast feeding provides very little protection against gastroenteritis. This impression arose out of visits I made last winter to countries in the Near East region, including Lebanon, Iran, Iraq, and Egypt. In some of these countries the whole picture of protein-calorie deficiency seems to be dominated by the tremendous epidemics of "summer diarrhoea" which occur regularly in the hot weather and which are followed by a wave of malnutrition a couple of months later—mostly malnutrition of the marasmic type. It seems likely that in these epidemics any infant is liable to contract gastroenteritis, often followed by marasmus, and that in such circumstances breast feeding confers little protection. The child of course, is usually given some other foods besides breast milk: it is living in a dirty home, in insanitary surroundings, and will pick up the gastroenteritis infection whether on the breast or not. In the Koran it is laid down that a child should be breast-fed for two years, and it is certainly the custom in Muslim countries generally for breast-feeding to be continued as long as possible. But, as I have suggested, any protection conferred by breast milk tends to be "overridden" in countries where extensive seasonal outbreaks of gastroenteritis occur. In other parts of the world there is plenty of gastroenteritis, but it seems to appear in epidemic form with special intensity in the semi-arid countries of the Near East.

Khan: Summer diarrhoea is a big problem in Pakistan. In the last three years we have seen over 3,000 cases in babies and infants up to two years of age (67 per cent or more were between six and eighteen months of age). Only 4 per cent were breast fed, 29 per cent were artificially fed, and 67 per cent were getting both breast feeding and artificial feeding. All the mothers said they were in the habit of breast feeding for two years or more, but when the infant is aged six months they start adding some carbohydrate, or tea or coffee. This shows that breast feeding does give some degree of protection.

We could discover no pathogens in 27 per cent of the patients, but the majority of them were malnourished from the beginning. So although diarrhoea by itself leads to some malnutrition, there is also evidence to show that malnutrition may cause diarrhoea. This leads on to the question of weaning diarrhoea.

Wright: It is curious that Dr. György's experiments were done on mice with *human* milk. In domesticated animals, particularly cattle, in the very early period of lactation the colostrum contains antibodies, which reduce the incidence of infections and the

mortality in calves. One would like to know what the effect of
their *own* milk was on the mice.

Brock: Dr. György has often stressed that what we call *cow's*
milk is food for *calves*.

Jelliffe: The question of infant feeding is a fundamental part of
the interrelated fields of nutrition and infection. Statistics from
various parts of the world confirm that the pattern of malnutrition
is tending to change (Jelliffe, D. B. [1962]. *Am. J. clin. Nutr.*,
10, 19). As Dr. Aykroyd said, marasmus is tending to appear more
commonly in association with diarrhoeal disease. This change
hinges partly, but not exclusively, on the question of breast
versus bottle feeding. For people in the so-called developed
parts of the world and for those in Africa or Asia who have
sufficient money and sufficient education, the arguments in favour
of breast feeding are similar. However, because of poverty,
lack of money to buy sufficient quantities of artificial feeds,
lack of education (but not of intelligence), and also because of
faulty home hygiene, almost certainly the vast majority of bottle-
fed children in developing countries are going to be given dilute
feeds, heavily contaminated with bacteria, with the consequent
downward spiral of marasmus and diarrhoeal disease.

Human breast milk, on the other hand, has a very considerable,
though partial, protective effect for the human infant. Certain
specific antibodies are present, at least enteroviruses, but the
main factor is probably an avoidance of the diarrhoeal disease
which I think is produced by intestinal infection.

This leads to the question of weaning diarrhoea. Professor
J. E. Gordon and his colleagues (Gordon, J. E., Chitkara, I. D.,
and Wyon, J. B. [1963]. *Am. J. med. Sci.*, **245**, 129) produced
this concept as a working hypothesis. As I understand it,
weaning diarrhoea is a multifactorial entity, produced by
cumulative insults during the so-called weaning period, that is
when the child is in transition from the breast to a wider diet.
The components that go to produce weaning diarrhoea include
enteral infection (very possibly with organisms that are normally
non-pathogenic for older children and adults), lack of immunity,
malnutrition, and also the age of the child (in relation not only
to immunity, but to the ease with which he can be precipitated
into fatal dehydration).

Enteral infection is obviously related to what goes into the
enteron, and breast milk is a clean fluid, putting it at its very
least. However, many communities have customs of feeding
children with other foods from quite early on, or giving the child
water, often contaminated and unboiled, or mothers may clean
out of the mouth with a rather dirty finger, and so forth. So a
baby is partially protected from enteral infection by breast
feeding, only provided nothing else goes down the intestine.

Diarrhoeal disease, or weaning diarrhoea, going on to death from dehydration, is undoubtedly the most common killing disease in the world. Possibly the best practical measures of protection are avoidance of marasmus by breast feeding, and of unnecessary enteral infection, where once again breast feeding plays a major role.

If the tropical child is breast-fed, one is not excluding the possibility of diarrhoea, but minimizing it by allowing the baby to get through the phase when diarrhoea is likely to be most lethal and most dangerous, by postponing the inevitable enteral infection until such time as the child is better able to cope with it.

Morley: I always get confused over this word weaning, and one can get equally confused over the word weanling. I had understood from Gordon's work that he was referring to the time when the foods begin to be added. For example, in West Africa mothers start to add food when the infants are aged four to six months, but it was when the child came off the breast, at 23 months, that frequency of diarrhoea reached its highest levels. If the weanling period is the whole period from the time of adding food to the age of 23 months, that is a very long period indeed. I would think it is more at the latter end.

Aykroyd: WHO is trying to define what is meant by "the period of weaning". I think that the term "weanling", as used by Gordon, related to the total period during which breast milk is being replaced by other foods, and not to the point at which the infant is finally removed altogether from the breast.

Jelliffe: I agree. This word weaning is too often used in a variety of imprecise ways. However, I still feel that Gordon's "weanling diarrhoea" is a most useful working hypothesis, and one which is worth investigating.

Brock: We ought to add to the survey that you gave, Professor Jelliffe, the concept that came out of György's work, namely the effect of the material fed into the gastrointestinal tract on the endogenous flora. Dr. György stressed that *Lactobacillus bifidus* was an organism that flourished in the intestinal tract of the child at the breast and which disappeared when the child was removed from the breast. Professor Gustafsson, can you say anything on this subject, which is obviously closely related to your paper?

Gustafsson: It has been well proven that certain factors in human milk influence the growth and metabolism of intestinal bacteria. We have been generally interested in the factors which might change the flora of the child or the adult, although we studied this in animals of course. It is not so easy to change the

flora as one would imagine. The flora is rather constant. Lactose
is one of the few factors that can be introduced into the diet that
changes the flora considerably.

Hendrickse: With cow's milk, one is introducing a beautiful
culture medium and this destroys the experiment immediately.

It is rather unfortunate that in 1967 we should still be dealing
with this subject at the level of impressions and opinions.
Diarrhoea unquestionably occurs at all ages, and may occur in
children who are totally breast-fed, but it is commoner in those
who are not breast-fed at all. In Ibadan, the incidence of
diarrhoea apparently increases to its maximum just about the
time that breast milk is discontinued, at around two years of age.
The organisms present in the stools vary considerably. We isolate
a recognizable bacterial pathogen in only about 20 per cent of our
cases. We have not been able to investigate the role of enteroviruses.

It does seem that susceptibilty to diarrhoea is related to
withdrawal of breast milk, but termination of breast feeding is
usually preceded by a period of progressive malnutrition. The
pattern of fluid and electrolyte disturbance in most of these
children is one of dehydration and "dilution", with low serum
levels of all the electrolytes. The explosive diarrhoea of the
well-nourished child, giving rise to hyperelectrolytaemia, is a
pattern we see infrequently and one which occurs mainly in the
first few months of life. The older children seem to have been
running down for a long time before the incident that actually
brings them into hospital. This experience is shared by many
people, and it seems that malnutrition is a very important
precursor of this actual incident. When we talk about the effect of
discontinuing breast feeding we are talking not so much about
the loss of protective effects peculiar to breast milk as about the
diminishing quantity of pure nutrients and the effect this has on
the child.

Vahlquist: Perhaps 80 per cent of babies fed on cow's milk
show signs of specific antibodies against cow's milk protein.
It is well known that the infant, especially, has the capacity to
absorb non-digested protein, so in itself the high percentage of
antibodies is not surprising, but it is surprising that this should
not have any ill effects later on. So far I don't know of anybody
who has been able to follow this up clinically.

I must agree wholeheartedly with Professor Jelliffe's
statement of the importance of breast feeding in the first two
years of life as compared with other forms of feeding;
nevertheless we should like to have some specific objective
findings from which we could clearly say that breast milk is
nutritionally superior to cow's milk. Dr. György's continuing
search for really objective findings is therefore highly admirable.

Professor Jelliffe also briefly touched upon the interesting effect of breast milk on the enterovirus in the gut. This seemingly is exerted in the intestinal lumen rather than by absorption of antibodies. If we could have a few more such definite facts to use for propaganda purposes it would be very useful.

Wright: Milk has been largely valued by those who look at world food statistics as a source of very good protein. The general view now appears to be that this can be readily substituted by vegetable sources of protein, including soya. Dr. György's paper indicates that there is something in milk quite apart from the protein that is especially valuable, and presumably this isn't present only in the very early (colostral) period. We have heard, too, about the inhibitory effect of a milk diet on malaria parasites, and mention was also made of lactose and its special nutritive value. This seems to raise a whole series of questions as to whether milk as milk may be especially valuable, quite apart from any question of protein content.

Mata: We have followed breast-fed children from birth to three years of age, in a highland community of Guatemala. The children experienced diarrhoea very early in life. The attack rate in the first three months was 4·5 cases per 100 person-weeks, increasing with age to reach 8·9 cases per 100 person-weeks at the end of the second year of life. Since diarrhoea is thought to be an infectious disease, we tried to obtain microbiological information by testing this cohort of children week by week for enteroviruses, adenoviruses, enteric aerobic bacteria, and parasites, and we found that the child is easily contaminated at birth. Thereafter, the child has a relationship to the environment mostly through the nipple, and he gets protection from virus infections through maternal immunity and from some protective factors in the milk itself. In spite of this, virus infections occur during the first few months of life. With bacteria the findings are different. The chances of the child getting shigella, salmonella and parasites are similar to their chances of acquiring viruses because the prevalence of all these agents is very high in the community at all times. However, we rarely see salmonella or shigella in the very early stages of life, which indicates that if such bacteria get into the host, they do not colonize it easily. Unfortunately, we have not studied a cohort of children that is not breast-fed.

The few cases of shigella infection in the early period of life are interesting. One persisted and developed into a clinical shigellosis in a child that was artificially fed. We have found two cases in the first six months of life, but all were short-lived infections. Later on, when the child is receiving supplements, shigella frequently persists for weeks or even months (Mata, L. J., Catalan, M. A., and Gordon, J. E. [1966]. *Am. J. trop. Med. Hyg.*, **15**, 632). Whether the failure of shigella to colonize in the first few months of life is due to a protective effect of the maternal milk, to factors inherited from the mother, or to the selection of certain intestinal microbiota, or a combination of all, we do not know. It has been shown that boiled human milk or cow's milk supplemented with sucrose or lactose has profound effects on the pH and on the relative proportions of the various components of the intestinal microbiota (Gyllenberg, H., and Roine, P. [1957]. *Acta path. microbiol. scand.*, **41**, 144). These observations provide a nice working hypothesis for further study of the human host.

Maegraith: I was hoping some paediatrician would define breast feeding. Professor Hendrickse used the very interesting phrase: "totally breast-fed". Often when we think a baby is being fed entirely on the breast in fact it isn't so. The point at which overt supplements are said to be given often depends on whether the information comes from somebody who works in a hospital or somebody who is actually working in a village. Even in the latter case, if the person belongs to the same race as the mother, the answer may be quite different. In north-east Thailand recently we discovered that infants whom we thought were totally breast-fed were in fact supplemented at the age of three days as a regular routine by the mother, who provided chewed-up banana from her own mouth—a very good source of infection. We should remember race and the way in which anthropologists can help us.

STUDIES ON PROTEIN-CALORIE MALNUTRITION AND INFECTION

W. WITTMANN*, A. D. MOODIE, J. D. L. HANSEN AND
J. F. BROCK

*C.S.I.R. Protein Nutrition Research Unit of the University of Cape
Town and the Red Cross War Memorial Children's Hospital,
Rondebosch, Cape, South Africa*

The kwashiorkor-marasmus clinical spectrum during the
first few years of life represents the severe and clinically
recognizable part of the effects of chronic protein-calorie
malnutrition (Jelliffe and Dean, 1959). On the iceberg
analogy (Scrimshaw and Behar, 1959), the much larger
hidden mass of the effects of chronic protein-calorie
malnutrition (PCM) in growing children is revealed in the
unsatisfactory morbidity and mortality statistics for
young children in developing communities (Scrimshaw,
1964; Wills and Waterlow, 1958). Although the interaction
of malnutrition and infection has become a well-known
concept (Scrimshaw, Taylor and Gordon, 1959), the precise
role of each has not been fully evaluated. It has recently
again been suggested that valuable information in this
respect could be obtained from long-term studies on
selected representative population groups (Expert
Committee, 1965).

The present report deals with the results of a series of
studies undertaken in our unit to assess some of the long-
term effects of PCM and to evaluate certain aspects of the
interrelationship of malnutrition and infection.

A follow-up study of kwashiorkor patients (first reported
by Moodie, 1961) has been analysed for the five-year

*Present address: National Nutrition Research Institute of the
C.S.I.R., P.O. Box 395, Pretoria, South Africa

period after first admission to hospital (Moodie, Wittmann
and Hansen, 1967*a*). Twenty-six per cent of the children
died in hospital (Table I). Infections contributed to death in
75 per cent of these and pneumonia or septicaemia was
most frequently incriminated. Nineteen of the children
subsequently relapsed with kwashiorkor on 28 occasions

Table I

KWASHIORKOR FOLLOW-UP STUDY

Total admitted	221
Died in hospital	57 (26%)
Relapsed	19 (× 28)
Died after discharge	16
Moved away	17
Follow-up, 5 years	131

(19 (× 28) in Table I.) During the follow-up period a further
16 children died and 15 of these died during a relapse.
Seventeen children left Cape Town and the follow-up study
was completed on the remaining 131 children. The results
of this study must be viewed against the background of
continued malnutrition which is known to have existed.

Compared with American standards (Nelson, 1959), a
large proportion of the children remained underweight and
stunted in growth during the follow-up period. At the time
of discharge from the hospital (beginning of study) a small
number of children had already regained weight into the
normal percentile range. After five years, however, 50 per
cent were still below the third percentile (Fig. 1). There
was no particular period of accelerated growth, nor could
the children be differentiated with regard to age of onset
or the degree of initial growth failure. Height was similarly
affected, so that the height:weight ratio appeared to be

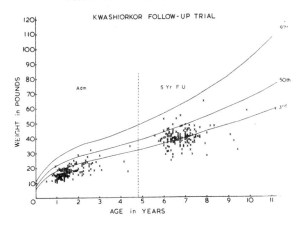

Fig. 1. Weights of individual children plotted against the Boston percentile lines on admission to the study and after five years.

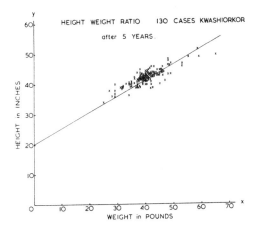

Fig. 2. The diagonal solid line ($y = 1·1875x + 20·130$) represents the theoretical normal height: weight ratio calculation from the Boston 50th percentile values. Each child in the study is indicated with an X.

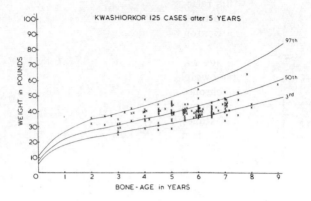

Fig. 3. The Boston weight percentile lines demonstrating weight for bone age as compared with weight for chronological age in Fig. 1.

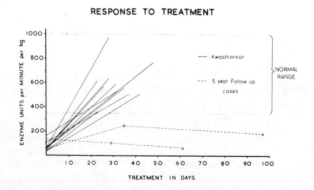

Fig. 4. A comparison of pancreatic enzyme output in kwashiorkor and prolonged PCM in response to treatment (Barbezat, 1966).

normal (Fig. 2). This ratio was not statistically tested but most cases fell close to the theoretical normal which was calculated from the Boston 50th percentile figures (Nelson, 1959).

In addition, bone age was retarded in such a way that the children had a normal weight and height for their bone age though not for their chronological age. Bone age was assessed from radiographs of the wrists and hands compared with American standards (Greulich and Pyle, 1959). If, on the weight chart, bone age is substituted for chronological age (Fig. 3) the weight shows an almost perfect scatter through the percentiles, in contrast with Fig. 1 where weight was plotted against chronological age. It is because of this proportionate growth retardation that chronic PCM often escapes detection. Whether or not growth failure here is going to be permanent, and what period of depletion would determine irreversible retardation, is not known.

From further work in Cape Town there is evidence that continued PCM in young children may leave irreversible damage in the upper intestine and pancreas. Gastric acid secretion was apparently not reduced by PCM *per se* (Wittmann, Hansen and Brownlee, 1967). Bowie, Brinkman and Hansen (1965) demonstrated lactase deficiency which failed to recover in all cases tested. More work is needed to confirm that it is indeed a result of PCM.

Berbezat (1966) investigated the exocrine pancreatic function in acute kwashiorkor before and after treatment, and in two cases of chronic PCM before and after protein repletion (Fig. 4). All cases of kwashiorkor recovered the enzyme output rapidly as soon as the serum albumin concentration improved. Both the chronic cases failed to improve even after three months of re-feeding. Do these two chronic cases represent irreversible damage from PCM or was the malnutrition conditioned by a congenital pancreatic defect? If PCM is responsible, the emphasis is on duration and not on severity of depletion.

Attention has recently been devoted to a hypothesis that chronic PCM might be a factor in determining the intellectual

backwardness of people in areas of endemic kwashiorkor
and PCM (Stoch and Smythe, 1963; Cravioto, 1963). Important as this hypothesis may be, we suspect that it will
be very difficult to put on a firm basis. Some of the difficulties are demonstrated from our findings in the kwashiorkor
follow-up survey (Table II). On clinical assessment there
were 24 cases with greater or lesser degrees of abnormal
behaviour. One was a spastic mental defective resulting
from hypernatraemia and probably a cerebral venous thrombosis. One child turned out to be a cretin. Abnormal genetic

Table II

ABNORMAL BEHAVIOUR IN 24 KWASHIORKOR PATIENTS

1 Spastic mental defective? cerebral vein thrombosis

1 Cretin

3 Mental defectives:	2 like mothers
	1 like 3 siblings
19 Abnormal behaviour:	3 low I.Q.
	1 normal I.Q.
	15 not yet tested.

inheritance was thought likely in a further three patients
where other members of the families were also affected. In
the remaining 19 cases (15 per cent), PCM could possibly
be incriminated but the contributory influence of home
environment, frequent infections and other factors also
have to be considered. This aspect of the study is being
continued by means of psychometry and electroencephalog-
raphy to determine the extent of abnormality and its
irreversibility, if not the exact cause.

The association of malnutrition and infection is also of
great public health importance in the subclinical forms of
PCM which are easily identified by the growth failure of
affected children.

The incidence of gastroenteritis in our hospital was

found to be highest in the underweight children (Table III). In summer 59 per cent of all patients in the lowest weight group presented with diarrhoea, compared with 16 per cent of the normal-weight children. In winter, diarrhoea remained an important presenting symptom only in the low-weight group. In addition the morbidity and mortality of gastro-

Table III

GASTROENTERITIS IN RELATION TO WEIGHT FOR AGE

	% of Expected weight		
	<65	65 - 80	>80
Summer			
Total patients	191	622	553
Diarrhoea patients	113 (59%)	235 (38%)	88 (16%)
Winter			
Total patients	134	387	626
Diarrhoea patients	38 (28%)	28 (7%)	33 (5%)

The incidence of gastroenteritis in an out-patient clinic during one month in summer and one month in winter (80 per cent of expected weight is equal to the third Boston percentile).

enteritis was influenced by the nutritional status of the patient. The figures in Table IV refer to a one-year follow-up study of severe gastroenteritis (Wittmann, Moodie and Hansen, 1967). The initial response to treatment was poorest in the low-weight children and they showed a great tendency to severe recurrent episodes of diarrhoea. Socio-economic circumstances in this group were so poor that one could not clearly define the relative importance of the multiple factors involved in producing this vicious circle of infection and malnutrition (Moodie et al., 1965; Wittmann and Hansen, 1965).

More recently a field study was undertaken for one year on a random sample of 30 children aged 0 to 3 years in each of four economic groups in a Cape Coloured housing estate for unskilled and semi-skilled workers in Cape Town (Wittmann *et al.*, 1967).

Table IV

GASTROENTERITIS FOLLOW-UP IN RELATION TO WEIGHT FOR AGE

	% of Expected weight	
	<80	>80
Total patients	64	37
Mortality	17%	8%
Poor initial response	55%	32%
Severe recurrent diarrhoea	69%	34%
Developed kwashiorkor	20%	7%
Total poor progress	71%	22%

Group A (Table V) was characterized by poverty, large families and poor social circumstances, all of which improved stepwise as income improved towards group D. The children in group A formed a striking contrast to those in group D. More than half (53 per cent) of group A children fell below the third percentile weight as against 17 per cent of those in group D. Recurrent diarrhoea, respiratory tract infections and multiple illnesses occurred most frequently in group A but diarrhoea was by far the most common disease encountered. The two most common findings on routine examinations of stools were the parasites *Ascaris lumbri coides* and *Giardia lamblia*. Ascaris was common throughout while giardia showed a stepwise drop from groups A to D. What role do these parasites play in the aetiology of recurrent diarrhoea and in the development of kwashiorkor and lactase deficiency? In Cape Town giardia was present

in nearly 80 per cent of children with kwashiorkor
(Barbezat, 1966) and about 65 per cent of them had lactose
intolerance (Bowie, Brinkman and Hansen, 1965).

Since economic poverty is so closely associated with
other adverse social factors such as overcrowding, poor

Table V

FIELD STUDY OF FOUR ECONOMIC GROUPS (30 CHILDREN
IN EACH)

Economic groups

	A	B	C	D
Income (cents/head per day)	14	24	36	50
Children/household	7	6	4	3
Overcrowding	83%	57%	17%	10%
Poor hygiene	90%	53%	47%	30%
Low weight	53%	40%	33%	17%
Recurrent diarrhoea	78%	60%	43%	27%
Pneumonia	20%	17%	7%	0
Multiple illnesses	53%	33%	27%	17%
Ascaris	87%	70%	77%	71%
Giardia	67%	57%	47%	28%

hygiene and social disorganization, one would expect that
a home environment which favours infection would also
favour the development of malnutrition quite apart from
infection. The one aggravates the other. Which is more
important? We can only offer a tentative answer from our
findings.

Table VI

DIARRHOEA IN RELATION TO WEIGHT AND ECONOMIC STATUS

Economic groups

*Weight groups**	A	B	C	D
I: <75% of expected weight	83%	75%	83%	No cases
II: 75 - 90% of expected weight	70%	42%	55%	33%
III: >90% of expected weight	87%	40%	31%	17%

*The numbers in groups I - III varied between 0 and 18.

Table VII

ILLNESSES IN FEEDING TRIAL (MEAN AGE 20 MONTHS) IN CHILDREN FROM VERY POOR HOMES

	No. of Children	*No. of Episodes*
Total	28	434
Death	4	
Diarrhoea	23	152
Pneumonia ⎫ Bronchitis ⎭	10	24
Suppurative Otitis	12	20
Measles	16	
Ascaris	16	
Giardia	17	

In Table VI the incidence of diarrhoea is studied in
relation to weight for age and economic status. Because the
numbers in the subgroups are too small no definite conclusions can be drawn. However, it can be seen that all the
children under 75 per cent of expected weight had a high
incidence of diarrhoea regardless of economic status. The
incidence was equally high amongst all the children from

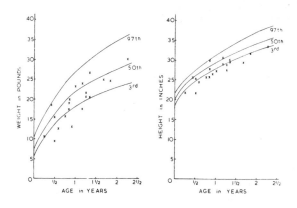

Fig. 5. Growth attainment with supplementary feeding. The weight
and height at the end of the study period compared with Boston
percentiles.

the lowest income group regardless of weight for age. In
each of the other income groups (B, C and D) diarrhoea
became less frequent as weight for age improved. The
incidence also dropped progressively with improved
economic status in the children who were above 75 per cent
of their expected weight. It appears, therefore, that good
nutritional status can "protect" a child against recurrent
diarrhoea only when the socioeconomic home environment
is reasonably satisfactory. Factors other than nutrition,
such as poor hygiene resulting in repeated infections, are
therefore also important.

The importance of infections under the most adverse social
circumstances is further demonstrated by a trial which was

undertaken to assess the growth potential of kwashiorkor siblings given a nutritious diet from birth.

Twenty-eight younger babies from 18 kwashiorkor families were given adequate amounts of milk and protein supplements from birth for a period up to 2½ years of age (Moodie, Wittmann and Hansen, 1967*b*). Infections, although not always serious, occurred very frequently (Table VII). Once again recurrent diarrhoea was the most common illness and respiratory tract infections next most common. Ascaris and giardia were found at one stage or another in all children over three months of age. At the end of the study some were of normal weight while others were below the normal weight and height percentiles although they grew significantly better than their previous siblings (Fig. 5). All but one of the underweight children had hypoalbuminaemia as well. At a comparable age only two of the siblings born immediately before the test children were above the third weight percentile and not one was normal in height. At least part of the failure of this trial must be attributed to the frequent infections which are apparently unavoidable under such home circumstances as existed.

The problem of the complex interrelationship of poverty, malnutrition and infection remains to a large extent unsolved. It would appear that to be most effective short-term preventive measures should be adapted to the needs of the particular group concerned. Under the worst social conditions control measures should be directed on a comprehensive basis towards improved socioeconomic status as well as the prevention of malnutrition and infection. Where the home environment is more favourable, "high risk" groups of young children can be identified by their growth failure and assistance should be particularly concentrated on *their* nutritional needs.

SUMMARY

The difficult vicious circle relationship between protein-calorie malnutrition and infection (especially gastrointestinal infection) has been re-examined. Evidence is presented that a low weight for age renders young children highly susceptible to gastro-intestinal infection. The pattern of diarrhoea may in addition be influenced by enzyme deficiencies of the pancreas and small bowel in patients with chronic malnutrition.

REFERENCES

Barbezat, G. O. (1966). M. D. Thesis, University of Cape Town.

Bowie, M. D., Brinkman, G. L., and Hansen, J. D. L. (1965). *J. Pediat.*, **66**, 1083.

Cravioto, J. (1963). *Am. J. publ. Hlth*, **531**, 1803.

Expert Committee (1965). *Nutrition and Infection. Tech. Rep. Ser. Wld Hlth Org.*, No. **314**,

Greulich, W. W., and Pyle, S. I. (1959). *Radiographic Atlas of Skeletal Development of the Hand and Wrist*, 2nd edn. California: Stanford University Press; London: Oxford University Press.

Jelliffe, D. B., and Dean, R. F. A. (1959). *J. trop. Pediat.*, **5**, 96.

Moodie, A. D. (1961). *J. Pediat.*, **58**, 392.

Moodie, A. D., Wittmann, W., and Hansen, J. D. L. (1967a). In preparation.

Moodie, A. D., Wittmann, W., and Hansen, J. D. L. (1967b). In preparation.

Moodie, A. D., Wittmann, W., Truswell, A. S., and Hansen, J. L. D. (1965). *S. Afr. med. J.*, 39, 498.

Nelson, W. E. (1959). *Textbook of Pediatrics*, 7th edn, p. 50. Philadelphia and London: W. B. Saunders.

Scrimshaw, N. S. (1964). *Ciba Fdn Study Grp Diet and Bodily Constitution*, p. 40. London: Churchill.

Scrimshaw, N. S., and Behar, M. (1959). *Fedn Proc. Fedn Am. Socs exp. Biol.*, **18**, No. 2, 83.

Scrimshaw, N. S., Taylor, G. E., and Gordon, J. E. (1959). *Am. J. med. Sci.*, **237**, 367.

Stoch, M. B., and Smythe, P. M. (1963). *Archs Dis. Childh.*, **38**, 546.

Wills, V. G., and Waterlow, J. C. (1958). *J. trop. Pediat.*, **3**, 167.

Wittmann, W., and Hansen, J. D. L. (1965). *S. Afr. med. J.*, **39**, 223.

Wittmann, W., Hansen, J. D. L., and Brownlee, K. (1967). *S. Afr. med. J.*, **41**, 400.

Wittmann, W., Moodie, A. D., Fellingham, S. A., and Hansen, J. D. L. (1967). In preparation.

Wittmann, W., Moodie, A. D., and Hansen, J. D. L. (1967). *S. Afr. med. J.*, **41**, 414.

DISCUSSION

Jelliffe: Nutritional dwarfing—or proportional growth failure—
is probably an important entity, and has been overlooked in
the past. We do not know exactly what the conditions are that
produce this end-result, but, as Dr. Wittmann has said, one
suspects that there must be an element of chronicity or prolonged duration. Certainly the condition seems to be common in
some parts of the world, and it may be much more widespread
than we realize. In the Lebanon, for example, E.F. Downs (1964.
Am. J. clin. Nutr., 15, 275) has found it to be common.

The syndrome poses problems in nutritional surveys employing
anthropometry, if the ages of the children are not available. It is
then extremely difficult to detect which children suffer from
nutritional dwarfing, as they are symmetrical, but "in miniature".

On an entirely different topic, work in Uganda has shown
that amongst some tribes, the Baganda for example, there is a
high percentage of congenital lactase deficiency (Cook, G.C.,
and Kajubi, S. K. [1966]. *Lancet,* 1, 725). Why this should be is
not known. Perhaps it is an adjustment to their habitual non-milk
diet over many centuries.

This leads on to the comment that cow's milk in my opinion is
not a necessary food for man at all. A liquid food, preferably
human milk, is required in the early months of infancy, but later on,
although cow's milk is an excellent source of protein, it is *not
essential.* This is evidenced by various communities, such as the
Hadza hunters of Northern Tanzania who don't have milk at all
(Jelliffe, D. B., Woodburn, J., Bennett, F. J., and Jelliffe, E. F. P.
[1962]. *J. Pediat.,* 50, 907), and by the excellent physique of
people in Polynesia (Jelliffe, E. F. P., and Jelliffe, D. B. [1964].
Clin. Pediat., 3, 604), for example, who had no milk animals
whatsoever, but who fed their children on breast milk and gave
them other sources of protein, notably fish, from an early age.

Dr. Wittmann, were the children with diarrhoea and those without
diarrhoea weighed after rehydration?

Wittmann: The weights have all been corrected for dehydration.

Garrow: These children who had kwashiorkor are presumably
selected from the poorer households and go back there, so it is
not surprising if they do worse than average once they get home.
In one of your earlier reports (Brock, J. F., and Hansen, J. D. L.,
[1965]. In *Human Body Composition* ed. Brozek, J., pp. 245-266.
Oxford: Pergamon Press) there was a parallel series of siblings
who had not had kwashiorkor. It would be interesting to hear about
these now.

In Professor Waterlow's unit in Jamaica we attempted to
determine the short-term prognosis for severely malnourished

children (Garrow, J.S., and Pike, M.C. [1967]. *Br. J. Nutr.*, 21, 155-165). Having excluded those who had overt infections, we expected that those who died or who recovered more slowly would be those with the signs usually associated with severe malnutrition—the underweight or hyperproteinaemic or anaemic children—but this was not so. Correlated with a bad prognosis were things like hypernatraemia, hyperkalaemia, and a raised bilirubin level. Of course these are conditions which are not necessarily due to malnutrition but which could equally well be due to infections which are not clinically diagnosable. I think that everyone will agree that it may be extremely difficult to diagnose infections among severely malnourished children. Apart from the long-term effect of infections preventing these children from attaining their potential stature, the damage in the short-term prognosis may be very great, even among children who have no obvious clinical infections.

Wittmann: The siblings during this study and at the end could not be distinguished from their brothers and sisters who had kwashiorkor—they were equally retarded in weight, height and bone age.

Hendrickse: Has a child who, for his particular height, appears to be well-nourished, although in fact he has this nutritional defect, a greater risk of infection?

Wittmann: As far as gastroenteritis is concerned, the answer is "yes". The children coming to the outpatient department referred to in the paper were divided into three weight groups and the highest incidence of diarrhoea and pneumonia occurred in those lowest in weight; the children of normal weight had a variety of other things, including minor infections and asthma.

Hendrickse: The implication quite clearly is that a child who has had this initial nutrition setback, even though he is subsequently well fed, is lagging behind not only in his physical development but also in his ability to cope with his environment.

Wittmann: But in addition we found a very strong correlation between progressive weight deficit and progressive hypoalbuminaemia, so I am not sure that they will lag behind if they are well fed.

Brock: We feel that the relationship between retardation of growth and hypoalbuminaemia is very important and that it certainly leads to a lack of resistance to infection in these children.

Hendrickse: There are two problems here: one child may be stunted and have hypoalbuminaemia in consequence, while another child who has been subjected to the same conditions but is subsequently well fed may not show a marked growth spurt and may still be small for his age, although he is in a good nutritional state. Is there any reason to believe that this second child has a continuing disadvantage in terms of his ability to cope with infection?

Wittmann: I don't think I can go any further, except to say that we interpret the growth failure as evidence of prolonged malnutrition whether the child had kwashiorkor or not. The *appearance* of the child is deceptive because weight and height are equally retarded.

Byam: Some children with kwashiorkor suffer lasting enzyme deficiencies in the gastrointestinal tract, and in both animals and humans gastrointestinal damage can be demonstrated to result from protein-calorie deficiency. Is there any evidence that the children with stunted growth have a permanent or lasting protein-losing enteropathy? This would seem to account for the hypoalbuminaemia in such children.

Wittmann: L. R. Purves and J. D. L. Hansen (1962 *S. Afr. med. J.*, **36**, 1047) studied this in kwashiorkor and were not convinced that there was any evidence of protein-losing enteropathy at that stage. During the follow-up period this was not investigated at all.

Maegraith: In malaria in monkeys the very notable slowing-down of absorption of amino acids could be made a good deal worse by the addition of either xylose or glucose to the diet. In the child that is developing kwashiorkor, with the bad balance between protein and carbohydrate, infection might make the absorption of the already limited amino acids a good deal worse, simply through this particular process.

Crawford: This malnutrition dwarfism can be produced quite easily in primates. A few years ago M. A. Epstein, J. P. Woodall and A. D. Thomson (1964. *Lancet*, **2**, 288-291) claimed that they had demonstrated a transmissible aetiological agent of Burkitt's lymphoma. This was in a monkey which had been injected with extracts of Burkitt's lymphoma tissue, which is thought to be virus-induced. D. H. Wright and T. M. Bell (1964. *Lancet*, **2**, 969-970), however, pointed out that this was not a Burkitt's lymphoma but in their opinion was an example of simian bone disease known to occur in primates in South America.

Some of our own work (du Boulay, G., and Crawford, M. A. [1967]. *Symp. zool. Soc. Lond.*, **21**, in press) seems to fit together now as a result of the discussion which has been going on here in relation to nutrition and infection. We have been looking at simian bone disease or what is sometimes called South American primate disease. With simple dietary manipulations it seems that one can stop growth and produce the most gross bone deformities, with collapse of the skeleton, pathological fractures, and teeth floating ih a rarefied jawbone. The evidence suggests that this type of bone disintegration is nutritional in origin. R. N. T-W. Fiennes, on the other hand, has demonstrated viral inclusions associated

with these bone disorders and he therefore connected a virus
aetiology with this bone-type disease (1964. ᴾroc. zool. Soc.
Lond., 143, 521-523; 1966. Symp. zool Soc. Lond., 17, 337-350).

I feel that the basic cause of this bone disorder is a diet
deficient in protein, minerals and oil-soluble vitamins but it is
also possible that under nutritional stress the disorganization
permits or encourages infection to take root.

The fact that Epstein, Woodall and Thomson (1964, loc. cit.)
thought the bone disorder in the green monkey was so like
Burkitt's lymphoma raises the question of a connexion between
Burkitt's lymphoma and the nutritional state. There is good
evidence that the Burkitt's lymphoma has a virus aetiology; if
this is so, is there a connexion with the nutritional status and
the success of the viral infection? This lymphoma is partially
susceptible to chemotherapy and if there is a connexion with
nutrition then this would be of importance in its treatment.

Professor Hendrickse tells me that Burkitt's lymphoma occurs
within a well-defined age group and is very rare in children
while they are still being breast-fed. The age distribution of the
disease may be related to antibody response but is sufficiently
close to that of malnutrition to make this question worth asking.
D. Burkitt (1964. In The Lymphoreticular Tumours in Africa,
pp. 80-93. Basle: Karger) comments: "There is an extreme peak
incidence at five to six years and not less than 62 per cent of
patients were between four and eight."

MALNUTRITION AND INFECTION IN ETHIOPIA

Bo Vahlquist

Department of Paediatrics, University Hospital, Uppsala, Sweden

Everyday observations in clinical practice clearly demonstrate that infections of an intense nature and perhaps long duration will markedly influence the nutritional status of the person affected. It is considerably more difficult, however, to demonstrate to what extent and in which way the reverse is true, i.e. how the nutritional situation *per se* will influence the susceptibility to infections, both with respect to the initial contraction of such infections and to their course and final outcome. (Expert Committee, 1965).

Experience from industrially developed countries has shown that even in subjects in excellent nutritional condition the course of the disease for many types of infections may vary widely. Thus for a bacterial disease like diphtheria and a viral disease like poliomyelitis a primarily infected subject may show all the variations from subclinical disease to a severe, even fatal course. If it is desired to use clinical observations to evaluate the effect of nutritional status it is necessary to study those types of infections which have a fairly consistent course in the well-nourished subject. One of the few widely prevalent diseases for which this is true is measles. Therefore the well-known observations of Morley at the Wesley Guild Hospital, Ilesha, Nigeria are all the more important and valuable (Morley, Woodland and Martin, 1963). Even if the strikingly high mortality figures in his series can never be said to depend exclusively on the nutritional status of the afflicted subjects—heavy exposure to other pathogens and lack of proper care certainly being causative too—they are nevertheless a clear indication of the detrimental effect of serious malnutrition on the course of this disease.

Our studies in Ethiopia (Agren *et al.*, 1966) have not been planned primarily to elucidate the problem of the vicious circle between malnutrition and infection. However, some of our observations may be of interest at this meeting and I shall therefore comment on them briefly. The detailed presentation of data will follow elsewhere.

MATERIAL

The Children's Nutrition Unit, an Ethio-Swedish project in the field of health, started in 1962. It is financed from Swedish (SIDA) and Ethiopian governmental sources. UNICEF and the Swedish Save the Children Fund have also contributed.

At five field stations in different parts of highland Ethiopia 2,830 children in the age group 0 to 10 years have been studied. The major stations are those in Addis Ababa and at Ijaji, a village 215 km. west of the capital. These both represent longitudinal studies which have been going on for more than four years, whereas the other three stations have been visited only at longer intervals, the information available thus being of a cross-sectional nature.

In order to characterize the nutritional status of the children many parameters, both clinical and biochemical, have been studied. Here only simple data relating to weight will be given as a background (Fig. 1).

It should be stressed that one special value of the data is that in each place they are derived from a very substantial proportion of all children living in that area, the attendance for examination being of the order of 75 to 100 per cent. On the other hand no attempt has been made in this part of the study to select a special group of severely under-nourished children presenting the picture of manifest marasmus or kwashiorkor. Selected material of this kind has been studied for other purposes in co-operation with the Ethio-Swedish Pediatric clinic but the results are not yet ready for presentation.

The pattern of infection and parasitic diseases has been studied by means of clinical, biological and serological data. For the purpose of this communication systematic observations related to microsedimentation rate, γ-globulin levels, parasitic infections and serological pattern will be presented.

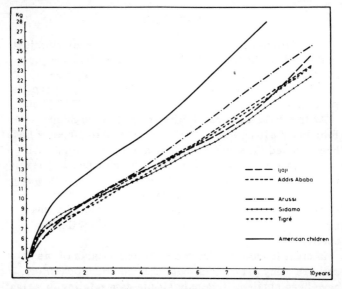

Fig. 1. Weight gain in Ethiopian children as compared to American children.

RESULTS

Microsedimentation rates. (Fig. 2). A strikingly high proportion of children exhibit sedimentation rates far beyond the limits given for children in Western Europe

(7 to 12 mm./hour), the mean values in several groups being of the order of 30 to 40 mm./hour. A careful study of

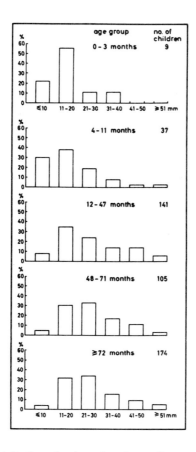

Fig. 2. Distribution of values for microsedimentation rate in Ethiopian children (village of Arussi).

environmental factors which may influence this value has failed to demonstrate that any factor other than the temperature is of importance, and under the circumstances given the effect of the temperature should usually not have exceeded the order of 5 to 10 mm. at the most.

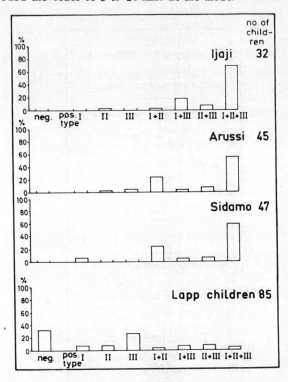

Fig. 3. Prevalence of positive aggutination titres for poliomyelitis. Ethiopian children 5-11 years old from three villages (Ijaji, Arussi, Sidamo) as compared to the situation in Lapp children 7-8 years old (Mellbin, 1962).

Gamma-globulins. The γ-globulin levels have likewise been found to be increased in a high proportion of the children, the mean levels at four of the five field stations varying between 1·4 and 1·7 g./100 ml.

In a selected number of children more detailed analyses of the four different γ-globulin fractions have been made

(S. G. O. Johansson, personal communication). These have shown that the increase in the electrophoretically determined total γ-globulin is essentially due to an increase in the γG fractions.

The reason for the frequent occurrence of increased sedimentation rates and γ-globulin levels should be sought in the accumulation of infections, since moderate, even long-standing malnutrition *per se* does not give rise to such changes.

Parasitic disease. The type and intensity of infestation varies considerably from one field station to another. Apart from high ascaris infestation in many areas and moderate hookworm and *Entamoeba haemolytica* infestation in some of the areas, the prevalence of notably harmful invaders is not very high.

Antibody pattern. Antibody determinations are an important addition to clinical and epidemiological observations since they may reveal previous subclinical infections and also manifest clinical infections which have occurred in the long periods between regular or irregular medical check-ups, and which have not been mentioned by the parents or at least have not been well enough described by them to permit a definite diagnosis. Of course the values noted in many situations give an incomplete picture if measurable levels of antibodies persist only for a short time or if booster effects through recurrent infections do not occur with sufficient frequency. With these reservations the following observations deserve mention.

Poliomyelitis. In Ethiopia immunity is acquired early (Fig. 3), just as in western countries, and probably in many cases while the newborn child is still under the protection of maternal antibodies. Hence cases of clinically manifest polio are very infrequent.

Measles. In this disease the difference from the situation in western countries is not so striking. A large number of the cases are overt, as observed in several epidemics occurring during the longitudinal studies.

With respect to other types of antibodies only a few brief comments will be given here. Contrary to expectation specific antibodies were rarely found for either pertussis or syphilis. Somewhat more frequent were antibodies against salmonella. Rickettsial antibodies were rare and so were antibodies against schistosomiasis.

Clinical tuberculosis as evaluated from tuberculin tests, is seemingly not very frequent among the children under study.

Malaria occurs quite frequently in one of the five field stations. Only in this area was a relatively high figure for the spleen index noted.

DISCUSSION

What, then, causes the high frequency of markedly increased sedimentation rates and raised γ-globulin levels? The causes certainly vary from one child to another but we believe that one important factor is the almost constant finding of skin infections, often pronounced (e.g. infected scabies, jiggers). As an expression of the frequency with which such infections affect the lower extremities, enlargement of the inguinal glands, often considerable, was very commonly observed. In addition chronic nasal discharge, conjunctivitis, and so on, should be mentioned.

A systematic correlation between the parameters for nutritional status and the observations of infections (past or present) has not yet been made on our material. However, even if positive correlations are obtained the problem will still remain of interpreting their meaning in a potentially vicious circle between malnutrition and infection.

For the time being, therefore, we have only been able to demonstrate in a high percentage of Ethiopian children the coexistence of widespread moderate malnutrition and a high frequency of specific and non-specific signs of infections. The true nature of this coexistence—parallel effects of unfavourable surroundings or causative effects in one or both directions between these two factors—has yet to be determined.

SUMMARY

Coexistence of malnutrition and infection is a regular feature in Ethiopian children. Some observations from the work of the Children's Nutrition Unit—a joint project between the Ethiopian and the Swedish governments—are given to illustrate this. The almost universal occurrence of raised sedimentation rates and the early appearance of antibodies against, for example, poliomyelitis is underlined.

Acknowledgements

The data presented in this paper are the results of team work within the Children's Nutrition Unit project. Much of the material in this particular presentation has been collected and analysed by Dr. Tore Mellbin.

The γ-globulin analyses were performed by Dr. K. B. Björnesjö.

REFERENCES

Agren, G., Almgard, G., Mellander, O., and Vahlquist, B. (1966). *Ethiopian med. J.* **5**, 5-13.

Johansson, S. G. O. Personal communication.

Mellbin, T. (1962). *Acta paediat., Stockh.,* **51**, Suppl. 131.

Morley, D., Woodland, M., and Martin, W. J. (1963). *J. Hyg., Camb.,* **61**, 115-134.

Expert Committee. (1965). *Nutrition and Infection. Tech. Rep. Ser. Wld Hlth Org.,* No. 314.

For discussion see pp. 126-134.

INTERACTIONS OF NUTRITION AND INFECTION: EXPERIENCE IN NIGERIA

R. G. HENDRICKSE
Institute of Child Health, University of Ibadan, Nigeria

Clinical and epidemiological experience and a mass of experimental data support the general thesis that severe protein malnutrition and generalized malnutrition increase the susceptibility of the host of many infectious diseases (Expert Committee, 1965). Data summarized by Scrimshaw, Taylor and Gordon (1959) lend strong support to this statement in respect of bacterial, rickettsial and helminthic infections but not in respect of viral and certain protozoal infections. Experiments summarized by these authors indicate that antagonism is the common and well-defined reaction in virus infections associated with nutritional disorders, and that malaria also tends to produce antagonistic reactions (Scrimshaw, Taylor and Gordon, 1959).

Our local experience of the interactions between nutrition and infection has been reviewed with special reference to the influence of severe generalized malnutrition and protein malnutrition on susceptibility to certain specific bacterial infections, measles (the commonest viral infection recognized in clinical practice), and malaria. The findings of this review are presented here.

INFECTION, NUTRITION AND GENERAL MORTALITY IN CHILDHOOD

A review of 1,685 consecutive deaths which occurred in the Department of Paediatrics, University College Hospital,

Ibadan between 1st July 1964 and 30th June 1966 showed that approximately two-thirds of deaths were due to multiple causes, and 70 per cent of all deaths were due to infectious diseases. The age incidence of infections was as follows: birth to one month, 66 per cent; one month to one year, 85 per cent; one to five years, 73 per cent; over five years, 51 per cent (Hendrickse, 1967).

Bronchopneumonia and "gastroenteritis" were the commonest non-specific infections encountered, but in a high percentage of cases it was apparent that the former merely represented the final insult to children incapacitated by malnutrition and/or some other disease. Measles was the commonest acute specific infectious disease causing death. Other specific infections which made significant contributions to mortality were malaria, tetanus, tuberculosis and pyogenic meningitis. The vast majority of deaths occurred in children who were poorly nourished, and in the age group one to five years more than 20 per cent of deaths occurred in children with severe marasmus or protein-calorie malnutrition.

The findings in this review of deaths give strong re-emphasis to the fact that in developing countries like Nigeria, high mortality rates among children under five years of age are principally due to interaction between malnutrition and infection.

NUTRITION AND SEPTICAEMIA

Although there is much evidence to support the general concept of synergism between malnutrition and bacterial infection, there is very little direct evidence that malnourished individuals have an increased susceptibility to specific bacterial infections. We have reviewed our cases of septicaemia to determine whether there is any correlation between nutritional state and the incidence of infections with specific organisms. Table I shows the distribution of 186 organisms of different types isolated during one year from the blood of neonates and older children in varying nutritional conditions. The following points will be noted:

Table I

DISTRIBUTION OF ORGANISMS ISOLATED IN RELATION TO AGE AND THE NUTRITIONAL STATE OF PATIENTS

ANALYSIS OF 186 POSITIVE BLOOD CULTURES FROM CHILDREN ADMITTED TO U.C.H., IBADAN BETWEEN SEPTEMBER, 1964 AND AUGUST, 1965)

	Coliforms	Salmonella	Pseudomonas	Proteus	Other Gram-negative organisms	Staph. pyogenes and other Gram-positive organisms
Neonates	17	8	6	1	7	10
Older children						
Well-nourished	8	15	-	-	3	9
"Doubtful" nutrition	8	14	3*	1	4	13
Marasmus	4	10	4	-	-	7
Kwashiorkor	8	6	10	2	2	6

* 1. Severe burns. 2. Renal failure. 3. Post-measles, bullous skin eruption, corneal ulceration.

(1) Isolations of coliform bacteria were most frequent in neonates but otherwise showed no remarkable variation between the groups compared.

(2) The Gram-positive cocci were fairly evenly distributed between the groups.

(3) Isolations of salmonellae were most frequent among well-nourished children and least frequent among children with kwashiorkor.

(4) *Pseudomonas aeruginosa (pyocyaneus)* was isolated only from neonates and malnourished children and was

most frequent in patients with kwashiorkor. The three children of "doubtful" nutritional status from whom this organism was isolated were all suffering from serious debilitating conditions.

Because of the well-known association of pseudomonas infections and extensive burns, it must be emphasized that pseudomonas infections in our kwashiorkor patients were not confined to children with extensive desquamating skin lesions. However, a number of patients with pseudomonas septicaemia developed distinctive skin lesions. These lesions started as circumscribed areas of induration in the skin and subcutaneous tissue which rapidly developed central necrosis leading to the formation of deep circular ulcers with undermined edges. They appeared to us to be the result, and not the cause, of the infection.

If we bear in mind that children with marasmus and kwashiorkor represent only a relatively small proportion of the total number of patients from whom blood cultures were taken, it seems apparent that these patients have a heightened susceptibility to most infections and a remarkable and peculiar susceptibility to infection with *Pseudomonas pyocyaneus*.

MALNUTRITION AND MEASLES

In Nigeria, as in most other developing countries, measles occurs mainly during the first five years of life and causes serious morbidity and appreciable mortality. Reported death rates from measles in West Africa are hundreds of times higher than rates recorded in Europe and North America at the present time (Morley, Woodland and Martin, 1963; Hendrickse and Sherman, 1965; McGregor, 1964).

Many factors contribute to the serious prognosis of measles in developing countries, but continuing experience of the disease in West Africa has fostered the impression that malnutrition plays a dominant role. The following observations are presented as evidence in support of this clinical impression.

(a) *Analysis of cases of measles seen in University
College Hospital, Ibadan*

In 1964, 1,224 consecutive cases of measles seen during
the first quarter of the year and 253 cases of measles
admitted during the previous two years were analysed
(Hendrickse and Sherman, 1965). Among the facts that
emerged from this investigation are the following:

Table II

SEX RATIO IN RELATION TO MORBIDITY AND MORTALITY
FROM MEASLES AND MALNUTRITION AT U.C.H., IBADAN

Source of cases	Male/female ratio
All children under 10 years of age attending General Outpatients	1:0·83
1,224 consecutive cases of measles	1:1·06
253 consecutive admissions for measles	1:1·18
118 deaths associated with measles	1:1·8
233 deaths due to severe malnutrition	1:1·44

(1) The peak incidence of measles occurred in the second
year of life but the highest incidence of serious morbidity
was seen in the age group two to three years. Serious
morbidity, as assessed by the need for special treatment
and hospitalization, was found in 17 per cent of one- to
two-year-olds and in 26 per cent of the two- to three-year-
olds. The serious morbidity rate in the three- to four-year
age group was also higher than in the one- to two-year-olds.

(2) Whereas males predominate over females in total
attendances in our general outpatients departments, the

numbers of males and females among children presenting
with measles are approximately equal. Total admissions
for measles are higher among females than males and total
deaths from measles are significantly higher in females
than males (see Table II).

These observations on the relationship of age and sex to
measles morbidity in our cases are at variance with the
generally accepted behaviour of the disease, and obviously
must be a reflection of some local factor which is capable
of influencing the course of measles, and which varies with
age and affects the sexes unequally. We believe this factor
is protein-calorie malnutrition, which in Western Nigeria
has its peak incidence in the third and fourth years of life,
and is more frequent and severe in females than males
(Table II).

(b) *Measles Mortality in Children Participating in a
Long-term Growth and Development Study**
A longitudinal growth and development study on two
groups of Yoruba children, one drawn from well-to-do
families ("elite" sample) and the other from poor families
living in a traditional environment ("Oje" sample), was
started in 1962 and has continued to date. There are over
200 children in each sample and every child has an
accurately known birth date.
The incidence of measles in the two groups of children
has been very similar. To date, 122 children out of 225
(54·2 per cent) in the elite sample and 148 out of 298
(49·7 per cent) in the Oje sample are known to have had
measles. There have been no deaths from measles in the
elite sample but nine children in the Oje sample are known
to have died of the disease. In three other cases, measles
appeared to have initiated the chain of events leading to
death, weeks or months later. The last recorded weights

*Being conducted by Dr. M. D. Janes, Institute of Child Health,
University of Ibadan.

of the children who died of measles are shown in Table III
and also in Fig. 1 in relation to average weights recorded
in our elite and Oje groups. (Weight curves obtained in

Table III

WEIGHTS RECORDED IMMEDIATELY BEFORE ONSET
OF MEASLES IN 9 FATAL CASES

Case no.	Age (yrs.)	Sex	Weight (lb.)	British Percentiles
32	3 +	M	24·69	Below 3
*78	2¼	M	27·25	31
279	1¾	M	21·38	Below 3
296	1²⁄₁₂	M	19·13	7
152	3 +	F	24·06	Below 3
179	2½ +	F	24·56	10
312	1½	F	19·81	7
321	1 +	F	15·88	Below 3
124	1+	F	13·69	Below 3

*Severely anaemic

various other studies in West African children are also
shown for comparison.) Not only are the weights of all
children who died of measles well below the "optimum"
for Nigerian children but the majority also fall below the
average weights recorded in poorly nourished child
populations in West Africa.

The weights of the children who died were, with one
exception, below the 10th percentile for British children
(Tanner, 1958); the majority were in fact below the 3rd
percentile. In should be noted that weight percentiles for
our elite Nigerian sample are almost identical to those of
British children.

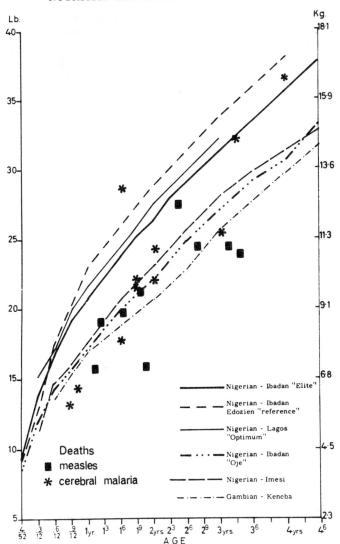

Fig. 1. Body weight in relation to age (boys and girls combined) in African children.

Morley, Martin and Allen (1967) recently reviewed information on 17,580 outpatient and 2,164 in-patient cases of measles gathered from hospitals all over West Africa. They found that the weights of children who died from measles after the first year of life were consistently below the 10th percentile for West African children. These authors were cautious about interpreting their findings, as the weights were mainly recorded during the illness, but they considered that their findings gave support to the conclusion that severity of measles depends to a large extent on the nutritional state.

From all the available evidence from our own studies and those of others (Morley, Martin and Allen, 1967; Morley, Woodland and Martin, 1963), it must be concluded that interaction between malnutrition and measles is strongly synergistic and that malnutrition is probably the major determinant of the serious prognosis of measles in West Africa.

MALNUTRITION AND MALARIA

Malaria is holo-endemic in Nigeria. *Plasmodium falciparum* is the dominant parasite and accounts for most serious morbidity due to malaria. *Plasmodium malariae* comes next in frequency and has been incriminated in the aetiology of the nephrotic syndrome, which is common in Nigerian children (Gilles and Hendrickse, 1963; Hendrickse and Gilles, 1963). There is also a low incidence of *Plasmodium ovale* but this seems to be of no clinical importance (Edington, 1967).

The indigenous population shows a remarkable degree of immunity to all forms of malaria during the first three months of life, but thereafter there is a rapid rise in the incidence of infection with *P. falciparum* and by one to two years of age over 80 per cent of unprotected children have acquired the infection. This high incidence persists throughout the early years of life and only declines significantly during adolescence (Bruce-Chwatt, 1952; Gilles, 1964). Infection with *P. malariae* also starts early and shows a slowly rising incidence to a peak of about 25 per cent at five years of age, after which the incidence gradually falls to below 5 per cent after ten years of age (Gilles and Hendrickse, 1963).

A high incidence of malaria in a population which also has a high incidence of malnutrition suggests that there is synergism between malnutrition and malaria. Impressions gained in clinical practice, on the other hand, suggest that serious morbidity due to *P. falciparum* may be less frequent in malnourished children than in well-nourished children. To test this impression a series of retrospective investigations of the interactions of malaria and malnutrition were undertaken. The findings in these investigations were as follows:

Table IV

RELATIONSHIP OF TYPE AND SEVERITY OF MALARIA
TO NUTRITIONAL STATUS IN 77 RANDOMLY SELECTED CASES

Type of malaria and severity	Nutritional state	
	Good	Malnourished
P. falciparum +	26	17
P. falciparum + + or + + +	15	3
P. malariae	5	11

(1) One hundred reports of significant malarial parasitaemia were randomly chosen from the records in our Department of Microbiology. The hospital records of these cases were then reviewed to determine the nutritional state at the time that malaria was diagnosed. Twenty-three cases had to be discarded because the relevant clinical information was not available. Findings in the remaining 77 cases are shown in Table IV. It will be seen that heavy

infections with *P. falciparum* were much more frequently
observed in well-nourished than poorly nourished children,
but infections with *P. malariae* appeared to be commoner in
the malnourished children. There were two deaths; both
were well-nourished children with *P. falciparum* infections.

(2) Autopsy records in the Department of Pathology,
covering a three-year period, were examined for confirmed
cases of cerebral malaria uncomplicated by any other
pathology. Eleven cases were found in which (a) the
diagnosis of cerebral malaria was confirmed both by
identification of parasites and typical histological lesions
in the brain, (b) there were no associated conditions which
might have contributed to death, and (c) accurate weights
recorded at the time of death were available. None of these
children showed obvious evidence of malnutrition but the
weights recorded varied from below average for rural
Nigerian children to above average for "well-to-do"
Nigerian children (see Fig. 1). It is of interest to note that
the pathologist's comments on the nutritional state of two
of the cases of *below* average weight were "well covered"
and "well nourished" respectively.

(3) Of 233 consecutive deaths in severely malnourished
children (kwashiorkor and marasmus), malaria was
definitely incriminated as a contributory cause of death in
only three cases. The anticipated incidence of malaria,
based on the total number of deaths due to malaria in the
Department of Paediatrics, would have been 16 cases.

(4) If there is antagonism between malnutrition and
malaria, the higher incidence of severe malnutrition noted
in females in our area should be reflected in a lower death
rate from malaria in girls than boys. Relevant sex ratios
recorded in our analysis of deaths in the Department of
Paediatrics were as follows:

Male/female ratio: in deaths from all causes between
one month and 10 years, 1:0·85; in malnutrition, 1:1·44;
in malaria, 1:0·65.

Obviously, the results of limited retrospective studies
of the type recorded above must be interpreted with caution.

However, each finding is suggestive of an antagonistic relationship between malnutrition and *P. falciparum* infection, and taken collectively they offer considerable support for our clinical impression that severely malnourished children are less prone to the more serious consequences of infection with *P. falciparum* than well-nourished children. The nature of the interaction between nutrition and *P. malariae* seems to be different but there is far too little information about this relationship to justify any comment.

The interaction of nutrition and malaria requires further exploration. It is difficult to envisage an experimental approach to the problem in man as it would appear that the nature of the interaction of nutrition and malaria only becomes apparent in severe malnutrition, or with heavy *P. falciparum* infections, and ethical considerations preclude experiments which expose subjects to such risks. It seems, thus, that careful clinical studies in parts of the world where serious nutritional problems and malaria are both prevalent will probably prove to be the main source of further information about the interaction between nutrition and malaria. Such studies are urgently needed as the interrelationship of the two conditions may have significance for public health planners in developing countries. In saying this, I am mindful of the experience recorded in the Bengal famine of 1943, when deaths from malaria rose to 202·6 per cent above the quinquennial average, a few months *after* famine relief measures were instituted (Ramakrishnan, 1954).

SUMMARY

Interactions between infections and malnutrition observed in the Department of Paediatrics and Institute of Child Health, University of Ibadan, have been reviewed.

An analysis of 1,685 consecutive deaths in children gave strong re-emphasis to the fact that in the group aged under

five years in developing countries like Nigeria, high
mortality rates are mainly due to interaction between
infections and malnutrition.

Data are presented which indicate that malnutrition
increases host susceptibility to certain specific organisms,
in particular *Pseudomonas aeruginosa (pyocyanea)*.
Findings are also presented which strongly suggest that
malnutrition is the main determinant of the serious
prognosis of measles in Nigeria. Interaction between
malnutrition and malaria appears to be very variable, but a
number of observations recorded in clinical practice suggest
that lethal infections with *P. falciparum* may be less
common in severely malnourished than in well-nourished
children.

Acknowledgements

Dr. P. Sherman assisted in the analysis of deaths,
Dr. H. Grant in the analysis of cases with septicaemia and
Dr. M. Janes in the analysis of those with measles. Professor
G. M. Edington made available autopsy reports on cerebral
malaria, and Professor S. Cowper supplied laboratory records
of cases of malaria. I am grateful to these colleagues for their
help.

REFERENCES

Bruce-Chwatt, L. J. (1952). *Ann. trop. Med. Parasit.*, **46**, 173.
Edington, G. M. (1967). *Br. med. J.*, **1**, 715-718.
Expert Committee. (1965). *Nutrition and Infection. Tech. Rep.
    Ser. Wld Hlth Org.*, No. 314.
Gilles, H. M. (1964). *An Enviromental Study of a Nigerian Village
    Community*, pp. 22-23. Ibadan University Press.
Gilles, H. M., and Hendrickse, R. G. (1963). *Br. med. J.*, **2**, 27-31.
Hendrickse, R. G. (1967). In *Colloquium on the Living Conditions
    of the Child in Rural Environments in Africa*, Dakar, February,
    1967. To be published.
Hendrickse, R. G. and Gilles, H. M. (1963). *E. Afr. med. J.*, **40**,
    186-201.

Hendrickse, R. G., and Sherman, P. M. (1965). *Arch. ges. Virusforsch.*, 16, 27-34.

McGregor, I. A. (1964). *W. Afr. med. J.*, 13, 251-257.

Morley, D. C., Martin, W. J., and Allen, I. (1967). *W. Afr. med. J.*, 16, 24-30.

Morley, D. C., Woodland, M., and Martin, J. W. (1963). *J. Hyg. Camb.*, 61, 115-134.

Ramakrishnan, S. P. (1954). *Indian J. Malar.*, 8, 89-96.

Scrimshaw, N. S., Taylor, C. E., and Gordon, J. E. (1959). *Am. J. med. Sci.*, 237, 367-396.

Tanner, J. M. (1958). In *Modern Trends in Paediatrics*, second series, pp. 325-334, ed. Holzel, A., and Tizard, J. P. M. London: Butterworth.

For discussion see pp. 126-134.

EFFECT OF INFECTION AND DIET ON CHILD GROWTH: EXPERIENCE IN A GUATEMALAN VILLAGE*

LEONARDO J. MATA, JUAN J. URRUTIA AND BERTHA GARCÍA

Division of Microbiology, Institute of Nutrition of Central America and Panama (INCAP), Guatemala

Evidence has accumulated, particularly from animal experiments, on the multiple interactions between nutrition and infection (Dubos and Schaedler, 1959; Scrimshaw, Taylor and Gordon, 1959). The existing data, however, are less satisfactory for humans studied in their particular ecosystem. To obtain information about the interrelationships of nutrition and infection in early childhood a field study was initiated in a Guatemalan village in February 1964, in which diets, infections and infectious diseases were recorded at short intervals to determine their association with the health and growth of children (Mata, Beteta and García, 1965). In this study, mothers were examined during pregnancy and their children were observed from birth until two years of age. Efforts were made to avoid introducing changes in the ecological setting.

The village studied, Santa María Cauqué, is a Mayan village of 1,200 inhabitants, 23 miles from Guatemala City, at a height of 6,500 feet. It presents an environment, family organization and social structure typical of pre-industrial populations, with high infant mortality (83 per 1,000 live births), high mortality in the age group one to four years

* This investigation was supported by research grant AI-05405 from the National Institutes of Allergy and Infectious Diseases, National Institutes of Health, U.S.A., by the Guatemalan Public Health Department, and by the Pan American Health Organization. INCAP Publication I-419.

112

(54 per 1,000 population of that age), and a high birth rate
(50 per 1,000 general population).

The community depends mainly on subsistence agriculture;
the only sources of cash are from selling some of the farm
produce or from working on a neighbour's land. Food
shortage exists because of primitive agricultural practices,
land shortage, and lack of other income. In addition,
traditional dietary practices account for a low intake of
food, most of which is deficient in good quality protein.

Environmental hygiene is poor. Water is from public
fountains or faucets and has high coliform counts. Housing
is deficient, most dwellings having one or two rooms, a fire
on the floor, and only one or two beds for the whole family,
which has an average of five members. Defaecation is
commonly on the ground around the house, there is no
adequate garbage disposal, and sewers, when present, are
open.

The village has a primary school of western pattern, but
with little impact on general education and learning.
Practical knowledge is obtained in the traditional way.

METHOD OF PROCEDURE

From February 1964 to February 1966, 95 live births and
11 stillbirths occurred in the village; 84 of the 95 were
recruited into the study. Of the 84, nine died, one migrated
and 29 were discharged either because of unsatisfactory
co-operation of the parents or to keep the size of the cohort
from taxing the field and laboratory capacity. This study is a
report on the resulting group of 45 babies, about half of all
those born in this village within the two-year period. At the
time of this analysis, 14 were less than two years old but
older than 15 months, and 28 were two years or older; two
died and one dropped out during the second year of life.

Weight was determined within 60 minutes of birth, then
weekly during the first month, and twice monthly thereafter.
A physical examination of the newborn was made within
18 hours of birth, then every week for one month, and

twice monthly thereafter. Additional weighings were made
before and after each attack of illness as part of the
medical control and care provided.

Dietary regimens were determined by weekly home visits
and the nutritive value of the diet was calculated (Flores
et al., 1960). No attempt was made to influence dietary
practices.

Frequent visits by the physician, nurses and field
workers permitted collection of weekly faecal specimens
that were processed in the field laboratory within one hour
of collection for: (a) isolation of enteroviruses and
adenoviruses: (b) identification of shigellae, enteropathogenic
Escherichia coli, and salmonellae; and (c) examination for
intestinal parasites (Mata and Beteta, 1965).

RESULTS

Growth of children in the first two years of life

Children of the village averaged 5 lb. 14 oz. ±11 oz.
(= 2·675 ± 0·311 kg.) at birth, that is about 1½ lb. less than
Iowa children (Jackson and Kelly, 1945). This standard
was used because INCAP studies have demonstrated that
well-nourished, healthy Central American children grow at
the same rate as Iowa children. Thirteen per cent of
children born in this community were premature babies,
considering both weight at birth and age of gestation. The
average weight curve for the series is shown in Fig. 1, with
growth up to three to four months of age closely following
that of the 16th percentile of the standard. Thereafter
weights departed from the standard, and increments from six
months onwards were progressively smaller than the
standard.

The progressive deterioration in gain of weight in the
cohort of 45 children is illustrated in Table I, where weight
deficits from the 16th percentile of the standard at three-
month intervals are shown. At birth, only two children had
weights at or above the 16th percentile, and most had

deficits of from 1 to 24 per cent. By three months of age, many children had attained the standard, for 30 per cent were then at the 16th percentile or better. At six months of age, however, deficits were noted more frequently, and at nine months, 68 per cent of infants showed deficits of from 10 to 40 per cent of the 16th percentile. At 15 months, more than 40 per cent had a weight 25 to 40 per cent less than the 16th percentile.

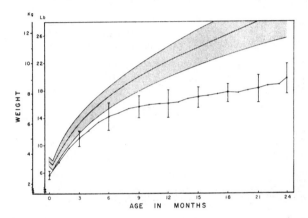

Fig. 1. Weight in relation to age in a cohort of 45 Mayan children. Average weight (dotted line) ± one standard deviation. Lines of shaded area are 16th percentile, median and 84th percentile of Iowa standard weight for age.

Factors influencing growth

Genetic factors and physicochemical and psychological influences from the environment affect the growth and development of the host, but are difficult to measure. Diet and infectious disease are two major factors which can be measured more readily.

Diet. All infants were breast-fed, almost exclusively, for the first six months (Fig. 2). Small amounts of sugar water, rice water or diluted coffee were given during the early months. Food supplementation ordinarily began at two to three months, with the administration of broths and gruels, and later—usually after six months of age—with solid foods, primarily tortilla, which is a sort of flat cooked pancake made of lime-treated corn. By one year of age, the child was usually receiving a supplement similar in quality to the diet of the adult, which consists mainly

Table I

WEIGHT FOR AGE OF A COHORT OF 45 VILLAGE INFANTS
(Santa María Cauqué, Guatemala, 1964-1966)

Age in months	No. of children	Children with weight at or above 16th percentile of standard*	Children with weight below 16th percentile of standard			
			1-9%	10-24%	25-40%	>40%
0	45	2	10	23	9	1
3	45	14	13	15	2	1
6	45	11	17	15	2	0
9	45	1	13	24	6	1
12	45	0	5	24	16	0
15	44	0	4	20	18	2
18	35	0	1	17	16	1
21	28	0	0	15	11	2
24	24	0	0	14	8	2

*Jackson and Kelly, 1945

of black beans, tortilla, meat, and vegetables, all in very small amounts. The amount of mother's milk contributed to the diet remains unknown, measurement being close to impossible under field conditions in the highland regions of Guatemala. The nutritive value of food supplements was calculated, and at one year of age represented only 17 per

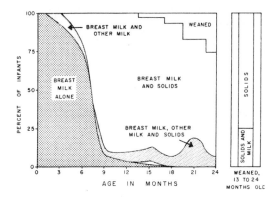

Fig. 2. Feeding pattern of a cohort of 45 children during the first two years of life.

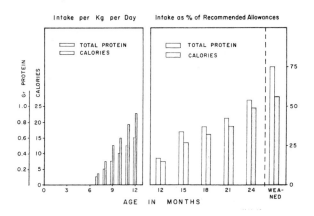

Fig. 3. Nutritive value of food supplements. Forty-five breast-fed children during the first two years of life.

cent of the protein and 15 per cent of calories in recommended allowances (Flores and Arroyave, 1966). Protein and calorie values of the supplement improved progressively with age, as illustrated in Fig. 3, but only to reach levels of 55 per cent of recommended calories and

Table II

BACTERIA AND VIRUSES IN MECONIUM AND FAECES OF CHILDREN DURING THE FIRST WEEK OF LIFE

(Santa Maria Cauque, Guatemala, 1964-1966)

No. positive in total examined	Group of micro-organisms		Day of life observed
5/5	Ciliform bacilli		2nd
	Coliform bacilli 10^9		
	Enterococci	10^{10}	3rd
	Microaerophilic streptococci	10^9	
8/45	Enteroviruses		1st and 2nd, one case 5th, one case 6th, two cases 7th, four cases

*Bacterial counts per gram of wet meconium or faeces.

75 per cent of total proteins in 12 infants of the series that were fully weaned before the age of two years. In similar rural populations, maternal milk becomes progressively insufficient for satisfactory growth from about six months of age; by 12 months it is definitely insufficient (Gopalan, 1956). It should be noted that supplements are not only nutritionally insufficient, but are also a vehicle for infection.

Infection and infectious disease. Contamination with faecal material from the mother or other attendants begins at birth. This accounts for the occurrence of enterovirus infections in the first week of life and for the rapid colonization of the intestine by bacteria, which reaches high levels as early as 15 hours after birth (Table II).

Weekly faecal examinations demonstrated frequent virus excretion during the first year of life often associated with

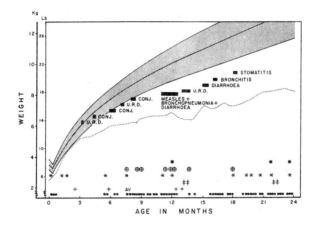

Fig. 4. Weight, infections and infectious disease in male child 168-24-08. Dotted line represents the weight of the child and shaded area is the standard. Length of bars indicate duration of illness.

U.R.D. = Upper respiratory disease;
CONJ. = Conjunctivitis;
   * = *Entamoeba histolytica*;
   ⊕ = *Giardia lamblia*;
   ✱ = Other parasites;
   ‡ = *Shigella*;
   + = *Staphylococcus pyogenes*;
   ● = Enterovirus;
     = Adenovirus;

illnesses. Some children excreted viruses in only eight weeks during the first year, others in as many as 26 weeks. These were mainly enteroviruses, although occasional adenoviruses were found. Pathogenic bacteria were relatively rare in the first six months of life. After six months, shigellae and salmonellae appeared, the former almost invariably associated with diarrhoeal disease. Parasites were found sporadically from the first week of life onwards, but colonizations were most persistent, particularly with giardia, in the third and fourth quarters.

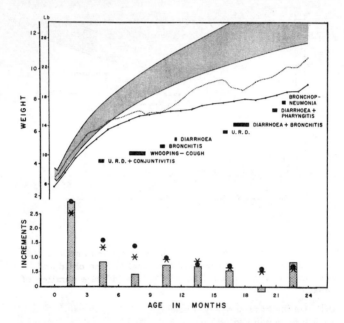

Fig. 5. Weight and infectious disease in male child 042-04-13. *Top*: Weight of child (dotted line) compared to average weight of the cohort (solid line) and standard weight (shaded area). *Bottom*: Observed weight increments (vertical bars) and expected increments according to standard values (●= median, ✶16th percentile). Duration of infectious disease in days is indicated by horizontal bars.

The frequency with which infectious agents were excreted in the faeces of these infants, and their association with infectious disease, is shown in Fig. 4, as illustrated

by one child of the series. There were repeated infections
by parasitic and microbial agents, frequently leading to
disease, particularly after maternal immunity was lost, and
host nutrition deteriorated.

Comparison of weight increments against expected values
in relation to microbial colonization and infectious disease
shows the impact of infection on growth. The weight and
clinical experiences of a representative child (Fig. 5) is
compared to the standard and to the mean weight curve for
the series. This child had several infectious diseases
associated with failure to gain weight or a loss of weight.
The weight increment during the first three months of life
was like the standard, but it was considerably less in the
second trimester, beginning at about five months of age
and related to conjunctivitis and upper respiratory disease
which lasted 16 days. The increment for the third quarter
also was low, being no more than 25 per cent of the expected
increment. During this period the child was ill with
whooping cough for 40 days. Increments during the two
subsequent trimesters were almost as expected, with mild
bronchitis for ten days in the fourth quarter and diarrhoea
for two days in the fifth. Deficient increments were again
observed in the seventh quarter, coinciding with diarrhoea
for 25 days and bronchitis for six days. Thereafter the child
gained weight more rapidly than expected, in spite of
several attacks of infectious disease occurring in this
period, but losses had been considerable and over a period
of months the child showed little indication of an ability to
achieve normal levels.

Although each case history showed the same general
picture there were wide variations in host response to the
same stress. Severity of infection is difficult to determine
on clinical grounds. Also, numbers of days of illness and
an expected effect on host nutrition cannot be determined
in terms of equivalence for the various disease processes.
These difficulties can be partially averted by using an
arbitrary criterion to assess the effect of disease on
growth. One used here is the concept of faltering, defined

as a failure to gain more than 0·5 lb. (= 227 g.) in a period of three months or more (Marsden and Marsden, 1965). In the present series, 33 out of 45 children studied during their first year of life showed falterings as here defined; one had a faltering in the second quarter, 22 in the third, eight in the fourth , and two had two such events in the third and fourth quarters. All falterings were associated with at least two attacks of infectious disease, diarrhoea and upper respiratory disease being the most common. Most cases of measles, severe diarrhoea, bronchopneumonia and tonsillitis were invariably associated with periods of failure to gain weight.

Of 22 children from whom microbiological information was available, all falterings without exception were associated with viral colonizations, usually of several weeks duration, and more than half had multiple viral infections. Two patients had falterings with concomitant shigella infection, and one with salmonella. Giardia infections were present in five falterings and dientamoeba in another.

The failure to gain weight during the first year of life was typically a feature of the third and fourth quarters, immediately after or before an infectious disease, but invariably associated with repeated illnesses and multiple infections of prolonged duration.

Interaction between Nutrition and Infection

The relation between infection and growth was measured by fitting the weight curve of the first 24 children completing one year of age by regression lines, and computing the number of days of illness experienced by the children with highest and lowest slopes for the weight curve. From the results in Table III it is evident that children with greatest weight gain experienced fewer days of illness, while those with least gain had the most.

Correlations for weight increments with infectious disease and diet for the same children were found to be significant for the second six months of life, when weight

Table III

NUMBER OF ATTACKS AND DAYS OF ILLNESS PER YEAR IN SIX
CHILDREN WITH GREATEST WEIGHT GAIN ($>b$) AND SIX CHILDREN
WITH LEAST GAIN ($<b$)*

(Santa María Cauqué, Guatemala, 1964-1966)

Disease	Children with greatest weight gain		Children with least weight gain		Difference days ill	
	No. of attacks	Total days ill	No. of attacks	Total days ill	χ^2	Probability
Diarrhoeal disease	12	100	11	170	19·3	<0·001
Upper respiratory disease and conjunctivitis	24	155	23	209	8·7	<0·01
Bronchitis and broncho-pneumonia	1	7	2	24	6·7	<0·01
Stomatitis and thrush	3	20	6	39	5·6	<0·02
Associated illnesses†	11	107	15	202	31·4	<0·001
Total	51	389	57	644	82·6	<0·001

* b calculated for second semester of life by the method of least squares.

† Two or more of the following illnesses: diarrhoea, upper respiratory disease, conjunctivitis, thrush and cellulitis.

was compared with total days of illness in the year and
when calorie intake at 12 months of age was measured in
the supplement. Also, with a multiple correlation analysis
of calorie intake at 12 months of age, total days of illness
during first 12 months of life, and weight curve slope

Table IV

CORRELATIONS FOR WEIGHT GAIN (*b*, least squares), ILLNESS
AND CALORIE INTAKE
(Santa María Cauqué, Guatemala, 1964-1966)

Comparison		*Correlation*
Weight increments for second semester-total days of illness in the year	$n = 24*$	$P < 0.05$
Weight increments for second semester-calorie intake at one year of age†	$n = 22$	$P < 0.01$
Weight increments for second semester-total days of illness in the year-calorie intake at one year of age	$n = 24$	$P < 0.05$

* *n* = number of children.
† Calories estimated in the supplement only.

calculated by the method of least squares for the second
six months of life, a significant correlation coefficient was
obtained (Table IV). Thus, a correlation of deficient diet,
high morbidity and poor growth was found, suggesting a
synergism between infection and malnutrition.

CONCLUSIONS AND SUMMARY

The diet, clinical experiences, and colonization by
microbes and parasites of a cohort of children was followed
from birth. The growth rate was adequate during the first
few months, in spite of an initially low birth weight.
Weight deterioration was apparent after three to six months,
associated with a progressively deficient diet, and an

increasing frequency of infections and infectious disease. The effect of infections was determined by comparing observed with expected weight increments, and by correlating days of illness with weight gain. An association between infectious diseases and failure to gain weight was demonstrated.

The enhanced clinical manifestations, increased duration of attack, and occurrence of multiple associated illnesses suggest a synergistic interaction between malnutrition and infection, which was supported by significant correlations found among poor growth, inadequate diet and high morbidity.

The precise time at which nutritional deficiencies, infections, and their interaction result in irreversible damage, and the magnitude of the insult necessary to induce that damage, have not been established for the human host. Studies of animals (Schultze, 1955; Widdowson, 1964; Dubos, Savage and Schaedler, 1966) show that certain early influences cause permanent stunting, even if animals are placed under adequate conditions at a later date. From this field study it appears that children living in the conditions described are affected within the first few months of life. The cohort will be followed to determine whether the retardation observed is irreversible.

Evidence has been presented on the interrelationship between infection and deficient diet, and on the effect of those factors on the weight of the host. Other stimuli, not yet studied, may be important even at an earlier phase of development. Among these, the following should be considered: (1) nutritional influences affecting the foetus and the newborn, such as deficiencies in the mother's diet and subtle or marked imbalances in the composition of maternal milk; and (2) early colonization by intestinal bacteria without associated clinical manifestations, specifically the establishment and interplay of the autochthonous microbiota.

REFERENCES

Dubos, R. J., Savage, D., and Schaedler, R. W. (1966). *Pediatrics, Springfield*, 38, 789-800.

Dubos, R. J., and Schaedler, R. W. (1959). *J. Pediat.*, 55, 1-4.

Flores, M., and Arroyave, G. (1966). In *Publicaciones Científicas del Instituto de Nutrición de Centro América y Panamá*, Recopilación No. 5., pp. 75-76. Washington, D.C.: PAHO, OMS.

Flores, M., Flores, Z., García, B., and Gularte, Y. (1960). *Tabla de Composición de Alimentos de Centro América y Panamá*. Guatemala: Instituto de Nutrición de Centro América y Panamá.

Gopalan, C. (1956). *J. trop. Pediat.*, 2, 89-92.

Jackson, R. L., and Kelly, H. G. (1945). *J. Pediat.*, 27, 215-229.

Marsden, P. D., and Marsden, S. A. (1965). *J. trop. Pediat.*, 10, 89-99.

Mata, L. J., and Beteta, C. E. (1965). *Revta Col. méd. Guatem.*, 16, 127-135.

Mata, L. J., Beteta, C. E., and García, B. (1965). *Salud públ. Mex.*, 7, 735-742.

Schultze, M. O. (1955). *J. Nutr.*, 56, 25-33.

Scrimshaw, N. S., Taylor, C. E., and Gordon, J. E. (1959). *Am. J. med. Sci.*, 237, 267-403.

Widdowson, E. M. (1964). *Ciba Fdn Study Grp Diet and Bodily Constitution*, pp. 3-10. London: Churchill.

Acknowledgments

The authors are indebted to Drs. John E. Gordon, Moisés Béhar, Joao B. Salomon, and Miguel Guzmán for valuable suggestions and criticisms. The technical assistance of Mr. Constantino Albertazzi, Mrs. Adelaida de Pellecer and Miss Ada Luz Colmenares deserves special recognition.

DISCUSSION

Morley: One point to be noted in developing countries is the median age for diseases, particularly droplet infections (by median age I mean the age at which half the children have an infection). In England and Wales in 1964 for measles this age was about $4\frac{1}{4}$ years, while in Glasgow in 1964 it was just over four years; in the developing countries it is much lower, about two years.

Similarly with whooping cough in England and Wales it is under
four years. In Massachusetts in 1945 according to J. E. Gordon
(1951. *Am. J med. Sci.*, 222, 333) it was 5·2 years.

In measles there are different kinds of rash. Rhazes in 850 A.D.
said that the rash of a dark red-violet colour is the bad and fatal
kind (see *A Treatise on the Smallpox and Measles*, Divisio
Morborum, Cap. 149. London: Sydenham Society, 1848). This kind
is often seen in Africa and communities which suffer from this
severe form are also those with kwashiorkor. I believe that
equivalent changes are occurring on all epithelial surfaces and
this will explain the laryngitis, bronchopneumonia and diarrhoea
which in the past have been considered ''complications'' but
which are part of this severe disease. This type of rash is
described in many of the old records in this country and I have
been able to get it from most of the developing countries.

The mean weight of 1,750 children admitted to hospital with
measles in West Africa was below the local third percentile for
children after the age of two years. The weight of the children
who died was even lower. The low weight of these children may
be explained by (a) measles being more severe in the underweight
(malnourished) child; and (b) the loss of weight that is so common
after measles (Morley, D. C., Martin, W. J., and Allen, I. [1967].
W. Afr. med. J., 16, 24-31).

In considering this problem of nutrition and infection we must
think of two very different things: (1) infection makes nutrition
worse (Scrimshaw, N. S. [1961]. In *Recent Advances in Human
Nutrition*, pp. 375-388, ed. Brock, J. F. London: Churchill), and
(2) poor nutrition makes infection worse. It is important to
separate these two in our minds. Two typical examples of the
interrelationship of infection and nutrition come from measles
and tuberculosis. F. J. W. Miller (in a guest lecture at the
Institute of Child Health, London, 1967) has shown that in India
poor nutrition makes tuberculosis a different infection. In measles
the mortality is 200-400 times greater in developing than in
industrialized communities. Whooping cough is different: it
certainly makes malnutrition worse but undernutrition does not
dramatically alter the course and outcome of the disease (Morley,
D., Woodland, M., and Martin, J. [1966]. *Trop. georgr. Med.*,
18, 169-182).

Garrow: Professor Hendrickse, you saw children with kwashiorkor
at the age of three to four years who had a high incidence of
infection. Are these children malnourished because they keep
getting infected or do they get infected because they have been
chronically malnourished?

Hendrickse: The study by Dr. Janes to which I referred has
been going on for $4\frac{1}{2}$ years; the data for the first four years are

now being analysed and I think she will be able to supply a
reasonable answer to that question. My impression is that the
malnutrition is the important thing.

Brock: What is the particular factor in Dr. Janes' study which
is going to answer this highly unanswerable problem?

Hendrickse: It is mainly because she has a prospective record
of the changes in two cohorts of children. We know their weights
and heights, and the incidence and types of infection that have
occurred. If we put them all together we might be able to get more
specific information.

Brock: Are these two cohorts separable from each other in
respect of nutrition?

Hendrickse: The "elite" sample is just above the London
average in height and very similar to it in weight. The children
in the other group are very similar to those in other village
studies done in West Africa, whose weights and heights are well
below European averages.

Jelliffe: Professor Hendrickse's results on malaria are exactly
parallel with findings in Mulago Hospital, Kampala, where about
10 per cent of the admissions to the children's wards were cases
of kwashiorkor—in other words, kwashiorkor was a common
disease. Yet, in seven years, no case of cerebral malaria was
diagnosed in a case of kwashiorkor. Conversely, in a recent
departmental review of thirty consecutive cases of proved cerebral
malaria, none were associated with severe protein-calorie malnutritio

However, this does not exclude the possibility that under some
circumstances malaria may be a considerable factor—a conditioning
disease—in pushing a child towards malnutrition. Anorexia and
fever, and possibly even the metabolic needs of the millions of
parasites scattered throughout the body, may play their parts.

Wright: The figures which Dr. Vahlquist gave for taenia
infestation in children in Ethiopia are surprisingly small. I always
understood that taenia infestation was rampant in Ethiopia,
certainly amongst adults, because of the practice of eating meat
virtually raw, and indeed that suitable taenicides were used which
grew locally. Why is the extent of the infestation amongst children
so small? Have eating habits changed amongst the adults?

Maegraith: With complicated organisms like malaria parasites,
the nutritional status may determine whether the infection is going
to be worse or better. It may well depend on what the parasite
needs. The diets short of para-aminobenzoic acid are very good
examples of this. Has anybody done similar studies to these
kwashiorkor studies in children who are suffering from marasmus
rather than kwashiorkor and are acutely starved? In both
P. knowlesi and *P. berghei* infection in animals starvation of the
animal suppresses the parasite.

Hendrickse: Dr. Ian McGregor recently informed me of his experience in Gambia. Originally he expected the very marasmic child to be teeming with malaria parasites, but over the years he has found that such a child is the least likely one to show very heavy parasitaemia. Our own studies include cases of marasmus and the experience recorded is very similar to that in the kwashiorkor cases.

The relationship between malaria and nutrition is obviously very complex and difficult to understand. We see folic acid deficiency precipitated by malarial infections: we heard this morning of the effect of malarial infection on the placenta and the infant. It seems that it is only at the extreme end of the spectrum of malnutrition that there is an antagonistic inter-reaction with malaria. In the rest of the spectrum it would appear that the interaction might be synergistic.

Maegraith: I would like to say a word about the effect of the nutritionist on infection. When we study these problems in the field, we should forget that we are doctors and remember the importance of the doctor, the agriculturist, the veterinarian, and the sociologist all working together on the same problem, particularly where it concerns children who have been moved from one environment to another. For example, a few years ago, to help nutrition in the north-east of Thailand, fish were put into ponds, rivers and lakes: these fish turned out to be the best possible secondary host for the liver fluke *Opisthorchis* and the incidence of infection has consequently increased in the area.

Jelliffe: An alternative approach to this problem may lie in lack of infection and its relationship to nutrition. A study by Dr. Robert Cook (1966. *J. trop. Pediat. Monograph*, 2, 13) in Uganda is in progress which aims to show whether lack of infection can improve nutrition on a community basis. This is known as the Ankole "Pre-school Protection Programme" (PPP). It is aimed at the comprehensive immunization of all Ankole children from 0-5 years. One object is to see whether these widely scattered rural children can be immunized against polio, whooping cough, diphtheria, tetanus, smallpox, tuberculosis and measles with fewer attendances than were previously thought necessary. The first immunizations for all these diseases are given to the children at the first attendance and so far over 100,000 children have been immunized. This type of immunization is being tested to see whether it protects against the infectious diseases, whether it is effective and safe for children who are far from well-nourished, and lastly whether on a wide scale it will improve the nutrition of the children.

Brock: Dr. Wittmann spoke about what I like to call a symmetrical growth defect or what Professor Jelliffe has referred to as nutritional dwarfing. There seems to be little doubt about the close association between this situation and the liability to infection. The question that arises is: does this sort of growth retardation indicate an existing state of malnutrition? We believe that serum albumin can be used to give a fairly reliable answer. We compared the serum albumin in patients with kwashiorkor during and after complete recovery, and in others who after partial recovery were put onto purely vegetable diets in order to test whether these were nutritionally optimum diets. We found a zone of marginal hypoalbuminaemia which we think is highly significant; in our laboratory the figure is 2·75-3·5 g. albumin/100 ml. serum. Obviously, these figures are only valid when they come from a single laboratory with a very special periodic check. We have been using exactly the same method for nearly ten years now, and it has been checked again and again, so we feel we can rely on these figures. When the serum albumin drops into that marginal range between 2·75 and 3·5 g./100 ml. we think the child is already very markedly depleted of protein (Schendel, H. E., Hansen, J. D. L., and Brock, J. F. [1962]. *S. Afr. J. Lab. clin. Med.*, 8, 23). More recently we have studied protein/albumin turnover with labelling methods. In three periods of marked protein deprivation in the diet there was very little change in the serum albumin but a significant change took place in the catabolic rate. From this we infer that one of the first things to be observed in patients submitted to low protein diets is a reduction in catabolic rate, and that this has already reached very significant proportions before the serum albumin begins to drop (Hoffenberg, R., Black, E., and Brock, J. F. [1966]. *J. clin. Invest.*, 45, 143). A number of people have questioned this concept.

Dr. Wittmann, did most children with nutritional dwarfing have marginal hypoalbuminaemia?

Wittmann: Yes, they had this fairly consistently. In children with gastroenteritis in whom the weight was corrected for dehydration, the incidence and severity of hypoalbuminaemia increased as the weight deficit became more severe (Wittmann, W., and Hansen, J. D. L. [1965]. *S. Afr. med. J.*, 39, 223). We found exactly the same in a group of children who were selected by virtue of either a normal or a low weight for age—just children in the street or at home. This is also true for the group of children in our kwashiorkor follow-up studies: the children who had kwashiorkor five years ago, their siblings, and the babies who were given dietary supplements from birth all showed the same thing. In the four economic groups in the field study, the weight deficit was by no means as great as this. There were only a few children below 60 per cent of the expected weight, so that we had a slightly better group and this type of correlation didn't come quite as clearly, but from group A through to group D there was a significant increase in the mean albumin value (Wittmann, W., Moodie, A. D., Fellingham, S. A., and Hansen, J. D. L. [1967]. In preparation).

Brock: This is the series in which a very positive association was found between the symmetrical growth retardation, hypo-albuminaemia, and experience of severe dehydrating gastroenteritis.

Mata: In our studies we have great difficulty in obtaining blood from the Mayan children, because there are taboos about bleeding, but we have been able to obtain samples at six-month intervals in many of them. In these, albumin values were within normal limits, even when there was a marked deficit in weight.

Jelliffe: The literature on this particular point, which I have reviewed recently (1966. *The Assessment of the Nutritional Status of the Community.* Geneva: WHO Monograph Series No. 53), suggests that there is not a very good correlation between the albumin level and weight deficit in mild to moderate protein-calorie malnutrition. However, your figures are so suggestive and interesting, Professor Brock, and the serum albumin test is so simple, that the problem should be looked into again.

Kodicek: We have made an experimental study of a specific deficiency, chronic folic acid deficiency, in which a breakdown in resistance to infection occurs in rats (Kodicek, E., Carpenter, K. J., Bradfield, J. R. G., and Sellers, K. C. [1955] *Voeding,* 16, 392-400). The chronic deficiency in rats was produced simply by producing first an acute deficiency with sulphasuxidine and then correcting the resulting agranulocytosis with small doses of folic acid so that the rats survived for up to 100 days and even for five months instead of the usual 40 days. During this period about a third developed lesions in the liver and spleen. The incidence of lesions increased with time, becoming high after 80 days. None of the controls which were given the same diet with folic acid showed this. On culturing these lesions we found in about a third of the rats *Corynebacterium pyogenes* which when injected into either rats, rabbits or mice was non-pathogenic. In a few cases we found *E. coli* or staphylococci. The question here is does the infarct come first and then invasion by the bacteria, or *vice versa?* We think it is the infection. One could argue that this is due to the agranulocytosis but acute deficiency of folic acid produces a much more severe lowering of the white cells than a chronic deficiency. We have no antibody titrations, but P. A. Little, J. J. Oleson and P. K. Roesch have found a lowering of antibodies in folic acid deficiency (1950. *J. Immun.,* 65, 491). What is interesting is that this chronic deficiency is probably the type that one could encounter in human disease.

Vahlquist: Does anybody know about the possible influence of severe iron deficiency on the susceptibility to infection? We know that infection can influence iron metabolism in the body very deeply, depressing the serum iron and also the transferrin and obviously causing a shift of iron from the blood to the tissues. In all probability this reflects some metabolic changes important in the defence mechanisms against infection. In a severe iron deficiency it is conceivable that these mechanisms cannot act in their usual way and perhaps the lack of enzymes containing iron might be detrimental. We know that iron deficiency is probably the most widespread deficiency disease, apart from protein-calorie malnutrition, in children of developing countries, especially in South-East Asia, e.g. Ceylon, where very few children under school age have normal haemoglobin values. This is a problem which needs to be tackled perhaps by animal experiments.

Maegraith: This is certainly very important. Experiments might be done in the area of oxygen acceptance, because with iron deficiency one might also couple copper deficiency; this brings in the cytochromes and lines up with the biochemical lesions we have already observed in malaria, where oxygen cannot be used.

Hendrickse: The evidence of magnesium deficiency in our cases of kwashiorkor raised the possibility that because of its importance in enzyme systems and so forth (Caddell, J. L., and Goddard, D. R. [1967]. *New. Engl. J. Med.*, **276**, 533-535; Caddell, J. L. [1967]. *New Engl. J. Med.*, **276**, 535-540) magnesium deficiency might well also be a contributory factor to the susceptibility to infections which these children show.

Maegraith: Magnesium and calcium are the two substances which are also known to suppress the activity of the mitochondria. Magnesium may be useful in kwashiorkor (Caddell, J. L. [1965]. *J. Pediat.*, **66**, 392).

Crawford: Professor Nicolaysen asked to hear more about the monkeys with bone deficiencies I referred to earlier. These disorders occur in both Old and New World primates in captivity and often occur because of an incorrect belief that all primates are vegetarians or because a vitamin D supplement is given that the particular species cannot use. The end result can be a virtually complete disorganization of the skeleton. A number of pathological fractures can be seen and there is also evidence of osteoporesis, osteomalacia, long-standing rickets, and secondary hyperparathyroidism. The jaw bone can show disorganization, with the teeth almost floating. This has been referred to as South American primate disease but it can be produced in a wide variety of monkeys reared on a poorly balanced vegetarian diet which

attacks them from several different directions by providing them
with a diet low in calcium (0·003-0·01 per cent), phosphorus
(0·003-0·01 per cent), protein and vitamin D (monkeys in captivity
seldom have access to sunlight or ultraviolet light, and there is
no vitamin D in fruit and vegetables; furthermore, some seem only
to use D_3 and not D_2). The combined effects lead to disintegration
of the skeleton. The skeleton recovers remarkably if the monkeys
are fed on a diet including milk, cheese and eggs. Inclusion bodies
have been seen in the thyroid association with these disorders.

Nicolaysen: Do they recover on diets containing calcium,
phosphorus and high protein but no vitamin D?

Crawford: They would get enough vitamin D from the milk, cheese,
and eggs. On this vegetarian-type diet the actual amount of
calcium present may be as low as about 0·003 per cent and the
same is true for phosphorus. One cannot correct the situation
by giving them meat which supplies protein but negligible amounts
of vitamin D. However, this may be because meat is calcium-
deficient and phosphorus-rich. We have not tried a vitamin
D-deficient, mineral/protein-rich diet yet.

The interesting thing is that it is so easy to produce this
catastrophic collapse of the skeleton in the small primates.
The same thing happens in Old World primates but they are bigger
and it is more difficult to produce this type of malnutrition.

Nicolaysen: Milk fat contains only 10-50 i.u. vitamin D per
100 grams, and the cheese given can in consequence supply only
a very small fraction of the vitamin D required.

Jelliffe: What is the protective diet consumed under the normal
circumstances in the jungle?

Crawford: People assume that because monkeys like bananas
they are vegetarians, but that is a complete fallacy. Although
it is difficult to generalize, in its natural environment a monkey
does not eat bananas, apples or carrots! Its natural food consists
of lizards, snails, slugs, insects, birds, birds' eggs, leaves, bark,
and berries–rather like the Hadza diet. These foodstuffs are
quite rich in protein and minerals compared with the cultivated
fruits and vegetables marketed in this country which are often
used as staples for captive primates. Even the young shoots of
green grass contain 11 per cent vegetable protein, but with a few
exceptions cultivated fruits and vegetables rarely contain more
than 1 or 2 per cent (McCance, R. A., and Widdowson, E. M.
[1960]. *Spec. Rep. Ser. med. Res. Coun.*, No. 297, p. 252).

Brock: This is relevant to many things that have been done in
the name of prevention of kwashiorkor. We have been interested
in whether it is possible to produce a purely vegetable alternative
to milk, with optimum nutritional value, and our experience has
been that it has not. Maybe we just haven't got the right

combination of vegetables in our mixture. This mixture produced good nitrogen retention, it initiates cure in cases of kwashiorkor and leads to a satisfactory improvement in the serum albumin level. But children put on this diet for a long period after they have been cured of kwashiorkor actually go backwards; and one of the things which definitely goes backwards is the level of serum albumin. The INCAP group has been the most successful in producing a purely vegetable-source alternative to milk.

Mata: The INCAP vegetable mixtures include yeast. Did all the cases go backwards on your vegetable mixture or just some of them, Professor Brock?

Brock: I think most of them did.

Nicolaysen: What was your experience in Ethiopia, Dr. Vahlquist?

Vahlquist: We tried products of this kind on a practical level, but we have not done any metabolic studies. We still include 10 per cent of dried skim milk so it is not really a purely vegetable mixture.

Mata: Our mixtures have been tested extensively in metabolic units at INCAP. Children who have recovered from protein-calorie malnutrition have been fed with this mixture as the only source of food, without deterioration of the nutritional state (Scrimshaw, N. S., Behar, M., Wilson, D., Viteri, F., Arroyave, G., and Bressani, R. [1961]. *Am. J. clin. Nutr.*, 9, 196). The mixtures were developed, however, as a supplement to diets that are not adequate. Occasionally, children with kwashiorkor do not recover with vegetable mixtures unless they have other recommended treatments. Physiological studies are now being done at INCAP on these cases. These studies will include an investigation of the associated microbiota.

GENERAL DISCUSSION

Wright: At the Ciba Foundation's 100th symposium (1967. *The Health of Mankind.* London: Churchill). I was asked to give a paper dealing among other things with malnutrition. As I said there, one of the great difficulties is getting adequate figures regarding the incidence of malnutrition, particularly in the less developed countries and therefore in the world as a whole. It is worth re-quoting from a WHO publication (1963. *Malnutrition and Disease,* p. 19. Geneva: WHO, FFHC Basic Study No. 12) which, referring to children of one to five years, states:

"Moreover, it is likely that a great deal more frank malnutrition actually exists and is lethal in this age-group than is recognized and recorded. A recent study carried out by members of INCAP has shown that a large proportion of the deaths of children under five years of age attributed either to diarrhoea or to parasitic infection were in fact due to malnutrition. Of the 109 deaths of children aged 1-4 years that were investigated over a two-year period, forty occurred in children with signs and symptoms of severe malnutrition, yet only one was officially listed as death resulting from malnutrition."

To obtain the statistical evidence which we need regarding the incidence of malnutrition there ought at least to be some method of indicating that, even if death itself was due to some specific infection, the latter had been very greatly influenced by malnutrition–i.e. that malnutrition was an important contributory factor. I feel sure that WHO would value ideas on how such statistical evidence on malnutrition could be more adequately obtained and officially recorded.

Mata: In an INCAP study by M. Béhar, W. Ascoli and N. S. Scrimshaw (1958. *Bull. Wld Hlth Org.,* **19**, 1093) all deaths of children under 15 years in a two-year period in four highland villages in Guatemala were investigated. Social workers were trained to recognize measles, whooping cough, diarrhoeal disease, protein-calorie malnutrition and other diseases; the records were examined and edited by physicians. Official causes of death in the children were compared with those obtained by INCAP, and striking qualitative and quantitative differences resulted. For example, 58 deaths out of 222 were attributed to intestinal parasites by the official registrars. Post-agonal migration of worms through the mouth and nose is interpreted as worms causing

135

death. None of these deaths were recorded as such by INCAP
workers. On the other hand, INCAP workers showed 40 out of 222
deaths where PCM was the main factor, and still others where
PCM was associated with infectious diseases, such as measles,
bronchopneumonia and diarrhoea. None of these deaths attributed
to malnutrition were recorded as such in the official statistics.

Hendrickse: If birth and death rates cannot be reliably computed,
accurate determination of the incidence of various causes of
death in the general population is virtually impossible. A few
years ago, in order to determine the principal causes of death in
the local child population as accurately as possible, we decided
to review weekly all deaths in the Department of Paediatrics at
University College Hospital, Ibadan. We found that even among
medical staff working in the same department, there are frequently
discrepancies in the causes of death recorded by different doctors
on the same patients. Even after a collective review of cases,
doubt often persists as to the accuracy of the diagnoses recorded.
Furthermore, in most cases death could not be ascribed to a
single cause and it was very often difficult to know which was
the most important cause in terms of initiating the illness or
determining the fatal outcome.

Very careful analyses of deaths in hospitals are urgently
needed, for even though they have no direct value in computing
general population statistics, they are valid indicators of the
major health hazards in the community. Reasonably accurate
evaluation of causes of death can usually only be achieved in
hospitals because in most developing countries they tend to be
the only places with experienced medical staff and the proper
facilities needed to achieve accurate diagnoses.

Maegraith: I entirely agree that bad statistics come not only
from villages and towns and the annual reports of medical
departments, but even from hospitals. It is very difficult indeed to
define the cause of death. Dr. Mata, how could you be sure that
40 of the children you described died from kwashiorkor?

Mata: The most overt signs in those 40 children were signs of
protein-calorie malnutrition. Other factors and possible causes
could have been unveiled if pathological studies had been done.
This is close to impossible in the field in a longitudinal study
such as the one just mentioned.

Jelliffe: A useful way of getting better statistics is to gather
information of three types. The first is from the direct assessment
of human groups: i.e. clinical signs present, anthropometry, or
biochemical tests. The second is from indirect assessment of
human groups, i.e. certain types of vital statistics, and data on
morbidity and mortality. (The latter may be from hospitals and
therefore not fully representative, but I agree with Professor

Hendrickse that they have a definite value.) The third is information on ecological factors which are responsible in part for the ultimate nutritional breakdown.

In regard to the last, it is useful to envisage malnutrition as a "camel's back disease" in which a child is loaded with one bundle of straw, if you like, after another, until one or another—an infection in one case, or a restriction of the diet for some particular social or cultural reason—ultimately produces the final metabolic breakdown. Among the ecological factors that one might look for in a community survey would certainly be the diseases which we now recognize as being most likely to precipitate severe PCM—measles, whooping cough and so on.

Brock: Has anybody any reservations about the observation that infection makes nutrition worse?

Nicolaysen: How does it make nutrition worse? Is it by malabsorption?

Brock: Professor Maegraith gave us one mechanism, a very important one (impairment of absorption of xylose in monkeys infected with *P. knowlesi*).

Maegraith: But have we really all agreed that infection makes nutrition worse? There isn't much firm evidence for this, although we all think so.

Hendrickse: Almost all children when they develop an illness tend to show a temporary arrest in weight, and most actually lose weight during infective illness. If arrest of growth or loss of weight, even if it is only for a week, is an indication of deterioration in nutrition then I think this is obvious evidence of the effect of infections in general on nutrition.

Maegraith: The fall in weight needn't have anything to do with nutrition. If the disease pushes up the metabolic rate, the weight will fall, and there are all sorts of other things which might cause this—for instance, loss of water.

Hendrickse: But if you push up the metabolic rate and the intake does not keep pace with this, then you are upsetting the conditions which afford optimum nutrition.

Maegraith: It depends what you mean by optimum nutrition. Are we not getting mixed up between metabolism and nutrition?

Brock: What about the possible different effects of bacteria, viruses and parasites, or are we lumping them all together as infection?

Maegraith: What happens in the infected host depends on the reaction between the parasite and the host as well as between the host and parasite, and I believe each has to be taken separately.

Hendrickse: Infection can influence nutrition in many ways. If a child loses his appetite or is vomiting and loses weight on that account, then obviously infection has acted against his best nutritional interests. I can't see any fundamental objection to that concept, unless there is any infection that improves nutrition!

Aykroyd: Some of the confusion in this field stems from
terminology. The very word "malnutrition" is extraordinarily
difficult to define; if you try to put into a paragraph exactly what
malnutrition means you get into all sorts of difficulties.

"Protein-calorie malnutrition" is a term that some workers
have used for a number of years. More recently the Joint FAO/WHO
Expert Committee on Nutrition (1962) has proposed the term
"protein-calorie deficiency." The terms perhaps differ in that
"protein-calorie deficiency" emphasizes the fact that deficiency
of calories and proteins, in varying proportions, underlies the
whole range or "spectrum" of indications from marasmus to
kwashiorkor; that is, it throws the emphasis to some extent on
what is eaten—on the diet. "Protein-calorie malnutrition", on the
other hand, is a somewhat broader term because the word
"malnutrition" suggests that other factors contribute to the
causation of the whole syndrome to some extent, in addition to
diet. Both terms are used almost synonymously nowadays. The
only attempt which has been made to express the inextricable
mélange of deficiency and infection is the term "weanling
diarrhoea", which is not very good in my view. We should try
to think of a term which would express the fact, which has
obviously arisen from our discussions today, that we cannot really
look at infection and malnutrition separately.

Brock: You don't like the term synergism?

Akyroyd: It helps, but isn't quite enough on its own. I was
thinking of a new term for the syndrome of "protein-calorie
deficiency" or "protein-calorie malnutrition".

Maegraith: The word synergism is used by Scrimshaw in exactly
the opposite sense to the way I would usually employ it (see
Expert Committee [1965]. *Nutrition and Infection. Tech. Rep. Ser.
Wld Hlth Org.*, No. 314).

The business of defining what we are talking about is the
important thing before us today, and I am not too sure whether we
can do it. Even weanling diarrhoea worried me a bit because the
meaning of the word weanling needed discussion. Mothers in
north-east Thailand, for example, provide pap to babies at the age
of three days, so it sounds as though weaning starts at the age of
birth.

Eide: A practical point concerns the possible reasons behind
early weaning. Reports from Africa seem to show that there is a
growing influence from industrialized countries that breast feeding
is not sophisticated. At the same time commercial advertising of
milk substitutes is becoming more widespread. Obviously when
mothers of poor families have to go out to work and leave the
baby with a grandmother and a more or less infected bottle, this
is one part of the story, which is a tragedy of course. But it is a

much worse tragedy when poor people with poor hygiene stop
breast feeding for the same reasons as women in developed
countries stop. How big a problem is this by now? What
measures, if any, can be taken to counteract this? Dr. Michael
Latham in his book on *Human Nutrition in Tropical Africa*
(1965. Rome: FAO) goes as far as to say that governments should
ban advertising to promote bottle-feeding, but this is perhaps
just one part of the problem.

Jelliffe: This is probably one of the most serious problems on
the paediatric nutritional horizon in the developing regions.
Basically a great deal of malnutrition in the future is going to be
what I term "commerciogenic". It is being produced, in my
opinion, by unethical advertising of commercial food preparations,
which there are no economic, educational or hygienic
possibilities of average parents being able to prepare properly.

Essentially breast feeding is a "confidence trick". If the
mother has confidence, she succeeds; if she hasn't the let-down
reflex is inhibited and lactation fails. The question is how to get
confidence back in these particular groups? Is it practicable to
ban advertising? I think this is very unlikely. Is it possible to
modify advertisements so that they are less harmful than at
present?—Perhaps. Can one try to exclude advertising from certain
places? I believe so. Health centre after health centre, with
public health nurses talking away about breast feeding, have on
their walls glossy calandars advertising proprietary milk
preparations. The milk companies also go round hospitals and
health centres in tropical countries distributing tins of milk to
"help out". These techniques are, in fact, low-cost advertising,
although not recognized as such by health staff.

However, a swingback is starting in favour of breast feeding in
some "over-developed" parts of the world. For example, some
years ago in Chicago the L.L.L. or La Leche League, started.
This is a group of educated American women who believe that
breast feeding is important for children in the United States, not
so much for nutritional reasons, but for the emotional development
of the mother and child. It may be useful, when trying to persuade
people in tropical countries that breast feeding is valuable, not
to talk about its nutritional value, cleanliness or economy, but
just to point out that if people want to be modern, or ahead of
the times, this is what is occurring in the United States.

*   *   *

Brock: Professor Gustafsson's contribution here today brought
out the important long-term or even permanent effects which may
result in the mammalian constitution from the form and the
intensity of endosymbiosis. The behaviour of γ-globulins in the

blood of germ-free animals and the contrast with control animals
suggests that the relatively high levels of γ-globulin in adults
throughout the African continent may be, as suspected, the result
of more intense exposure to micro-organismal antigens. We hope
some day to know whether or not the relatively low serum albumins
in the same people reflect relative dietary protein deficiency.

In the field of long-term or permanent effects of early environmental exposure we must remember that the antibody-producing
mechanisms of the reticuloendothelial system, to a greater extent
even than the brain, have to "remember" what happened in
childhood.

The two papers on the effects of malarial parasites tie in
closely. It seems likely that placental malaria affects the human
constitution *in utero* in spite of the apparent placental barrier of
the parasite.

The latter discussions tended to concentrate heavily on a more
limited aspect of our general title: I refer to the subject of the
"synergistic" or "vicious circle" relationship between malnutrition
and bacterial infection as exemplified in the clinical spectrum of
protein-calorie malnutrition in young children. Our programme was
indeed "set" towards such a concentration by the titles under
which contributions were requested; there is no doubt of the
world-wide practical significance of the subject. (Wittmann, W.,
Moodie, A. D., Fellingham, S. A. and Hansen, J. D. L. [1967].
S. Afr. med. J., **41**, 664-682).

But as biologists I think we have failed to maintain the breadth
of interest which the title of our meeting suggested. I would like
to have seen post-weaning gastroenteritis discussed against the
wider subject of the total interaction, from conception throughout
life, between favourable and unfavourable environment and the
genome. How far is the pattern of gastroenteritis in infancy and
childhood related to birth weight and a variety of intrauterine
influences? How far does it in turn determine, through the
"memory" of the antibody mechanisms, the later "constitutional"
reactions to infection? For example, widely differing diseases
appear to result, in different human individuals, from invasion of
the naspharynx by a single antigenic strain of streptococcus.

Our first three papers and discussions gave us some very
valuable, and I think new, clues which we failed to exploit in
our later discussions.

I am sure there will have to be many more discussions on the
subject of nutrition and infection before we come to ordered
conclusions on this subject. May I just say to Professor
Nicolaysen: we hope that you have enjoyed your day.

INDEX

141

Printed in Great Britain by
Spottiswoode, Ballantyne & Co. Ltd., London and Colchester
by offset litho from 'Colprint'